June 2012 - Still in print.
       oop. 9/14
Jan 2023 - OOP

$51. 05

Visit our website

to find out about other books from Mosby
and other Harcourt Health Sciences imprints

Register free at
www.harcourt-international.com

and you will get

- the latest information on new books, journals and electronic products in your chosen subject areas

- the choice of e-mail or post alerts or both, when there are any new books in your chosen areas

- news of special offers and promotions

- information about products from all Harcourt Health Sciences imprints including Baillière Tindall, Churchill Livingstone, Mosby and W. B. Saunders

You will also find an easily searchable catalogue, online ordering, information on our extensive list of journals...and much more!

Visit the Harcourt Health Sciences website today!

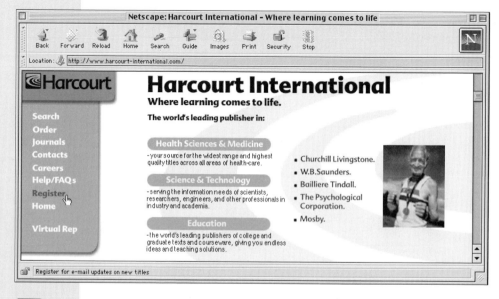

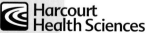

Safety at Scene

For Mosby:

Senior Commissioning Editor: Ninette Premdas
Project Manager: Jane Shanks
Design Direction: George Ajayi

Safety at Scene
A Manual for Paramedics and Immediate Care Doctors

Vic Calland OStJ MRCGP ChB DRCOG DipIMC RCS(Ed)
Immediate Care Doctor, Med-ALERT; Honorary Medical Officer,
Lancashire Ambulance Service NHS Trust, UK

Foreword by

Iain McNeil MB ChB MRCGP DipIMC RCS(Ed) DRCOG DFFP DIAEMD
Chairman, BASICS (British Association for Immediate Care), Ipswich, UK

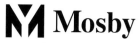 Mosby

EDINBURGH LONDON NEW YORK PHILADELPHIA ST LOUIS SYDNEY TORONTO 2000

MOSBY
An imprint of Harcourt Publishers Limited

© Harcourt Publishers Limited 2000

First published 2000

0 7234 3199 X

British Library Cataloguing in Publication Data
A catalogue record for this book is available from the British Library

Library of Congress Cataloging in Publication Data
A catalog record for this book is available from the Library of Congress

Note
Medical knowledge is constantly changing. As new information becomes available, changes in treatment, procedures, equipment and the use of drugs become necessary. The author and the publishers have taken care to ensure that the information given in this text is accurate and up to date. However, readers are strongly advised to confirm that the information, especially with regard to drug usage, complies with the latest legislation and standards of practice.

The
publisher's
policy is to use
**paper manufactured
from sustainable forests**

Printed in China

Contents

Foreword

The mantra 'Safety, Gloves, ABC' is one that all those who work in the pre-hospital field should never forget. Yet it is forgotten all too often and rescuers become the victims. It is true to say that ours is a dangerous business, but most accidents that happen to rescuers occur through ignorance or carelessness. Simple things can make all the difference to one's safety – the wearing of a hard hat or gloves, the correct assessment for danger in a collapsed building, the recognition of an evacuation signal – yet I often see seasoned emergency workers ignore all the dangers and fail to take simple precautions. Brave? Maybe. Foolhardy? Definitely. How many of our colleagues have contracted infectious diseases, or been injured from falling masonry or cut by debris, all because they were too engrossed in the job or careless to look after themselves?

I talk as though I am perfect – but I most certainly am not! I have dealt with casualties covered in blood without protecting myself with gloves – how foolish! And I have entered a collapsed building without a hard hat – fortunately to be given one by a sensible paramedic who undoubtedly saved my life as a few minutes later the building collapsed onto the rescuers, all of whom were fortunately unharmed – how lucky! I have, however, learned from my mistakes and have always worn a hard hat since – despite the heat and discomfort. I have felt the fear when, exactly one year ago today as I write this foreword, the evacuation whistle blew whilst I was working deep within a building collapsed by earthquakes that was being shaken by aftershocks. I know now how fast I can run!

But how I wish I had then the knowledge that is contained within this book. For with it I, and many of my colleagues, would not have made some of the silly mistakes that put ourselves and perhaps others at risk.

Despite the fact that safety should always come first – of self, then scene and then of the casualty – there are few ways that the paramedic and immediate care doctor and nurses can gain insight to some of the less commonly encountered dangers that present in their jobs. There are few books or articles that adequately address the myriad of situations that one might encounter.

This book goes a long way to addressing that problem. Within its covers you are led through the common dangers that are met and then advised how to avoid them or deal with them. Of particular note is a section that covers the various ways that a car can be demolished by the fire services. Another uniquely helpful section covers the problems that one might encounter where 'people affect safety'. This covers for example such situations as civil disorder, attack by mobs and entering crowds during disturbances: things that we are increasingly expected to do, often on our own and for which we have had little or no training.

This book is a 'must read' for immediate care doctors, nurses and paramedics and sits, in my opinion, alongside such publications as John Eaton's *Essentials in Immediate Care* and Nancy Caroline's *Emergency Care in the Streets*. It represents a major step forward in the protection of *our* lives. Read it from cover to cover and then read it again.

Ipswich 2000   Iain McNeil

REFERENCES

Eaton C J 1999 Essentials of immediate medical care. Churchill Livingstone, Edinburgh
Caroline N 1995 Emergency care in the streets. Lippincott Williams and Wilkins, London

Preface

In 1994 I was approached by the Lancashire Fire Brigade International Training Centre to talk to firefighters on their 'Crew Command' course. This course is primarily for leading firefighters, who would be expected to be in charge of an appliance and its crew. I was asked to explain the role of the immediate care doctor at the road accident scene.

As this course was covering subjects that I had never learnt about, and only watched happen around me in the six years I had been attending accidents, I asked if I could sit in on the two days dedicated to road traffic accidents. By the end of those two days I had learnt an enormous amount, and so had the firefighters. I was invited back and have since become a regular lecturer at the Centre, still attending every course for the full two days. My colleagues in Med-ALERT (the Lancashire Immediate Care scheme) also attended at least one course, and we were the first BASICS (British Association for Immediate Care) scheme in the country to make training with firefighters compulsory before going on the road.

In 1996 the instructors at the Centre asked if there was any training that they could give Med-ALERT in acknowledgement of the input we had provided for them. As a result the 'Safety at Scene' course was devised. The first course ran in the summer of 1997, attended by 13 doctors and Lancashire paramedics. It was an amazing success and prompted the Centre to run the course as a recognised subject. It is the first and so far the only course that specialises in teaching the safety concepts inherent in firefighter training to the other personnel who may be involved at an emergency.

In 1998 six 'Safety at Scene' courses ran, with people attending from all over the country and also from British Army bases overseas. The course has received higher ratings from students than almost any other that the Centre has run; this success has led to the publication of this manual.

I would like to make it clear that I cannot pretend to know as much about any of the subjects within this book as the experts in the relevant fields. The manual is no substitute for attending specialist courses and studying specialist books, a selection of which are listed in the further reading list at the end of the book. However, being a generalist by training, I am aware that many people who undertake emergency service duties do not have the benefit of the fire service safety discipline. I have therefore tried to cover the subjects with enough information to enable them to recognise the dangers and to have a basic idea of how to avoid them.

During the development of this book, because it is the first in its field, I was asked if it was going to be the 'definitive text of scene safety'. It is not. Safety is such a complex subject that there is no single book, nor even an entire library, that covers all aspects of the issue. It was suggested that if I produced lists of things to be done at any particular incident, then it would be a valuable 'on scene' text. I believe that reading this type of material at scene is far too late. By the time you receive 'the shout' your knowledge, skills and attitudes should all be focused on staying in one piece to enjoy your own life.

While a lot can be learnt from reading the manual, it is no substitute for attending a course. No manual can give its reader the experience gained from actually using fire extinguishers, ropes and cutting equipment. 'Safety at Scene' is the kind of course that must, and will, evolve as risks change, and so not only should you attend a course, but you should consider re-attending regularly. It is, after all, a course designed to keep you alive and safe.

Every situation is different, and to follow blindly what is only intended to be a guide is as dangerous as assuming that the advice within the manual does not apply. The human machine has proved extraordinarily adaptable on this planet, not because of its strengths, or the benign nature of its environment, for it possesses neither of these. It has succeeded over adversity because it uses its greatest attribute, its brain.

Your safety depends not on brute force, unquestioned attitudes or unrestrained emotions. It depends entirely upon your ability to use your knowledge and skills to determine the most logical way to resolve the situations you will face.

Preston 2000   V. Calland

Acknowledgements

It will be obvious as you read through this manual that a considerable amount of the knowledge within it has come from the Lancashire Fire and Rescue Service Training Centre. They in their turn have leant heavily upon the *Manual of Firemanship* (HM Fire Inspectorate/Home Office 1967–present), which has been the bible of the fire service for the last 30 years or so. Some of the ideas should be attributed to the numerous firefighters and paramedics with whom I have worked over the years, but it is not just these services that have contributed. Elements of the content are based on Royal Life Saving Society manuals, St John Ambulance manuals, diver training manuals, books on sailing, mountain leadership books, 'Safety at Scene' course participants and many, many more sources.

It is difficult to be original in a field where the training is not only didactic but also has to synchronise with declared policies of other organisations. How can an author explain the emergency procedures of the London Underground without drawing heavily from their own safety manual?

In particular I would like to thank Station Officer Kevin Gibson, who has patiently answered my questions, encouraged me to continue and, most importantly, proof-read the manuscript for me. I would also like to thank Rob Walmsley for the considerable amount of knowledge he has given me on rescue technique.

1

Basic principles of safety

Paramedics, immediate care doctors and police officers take time and money to train. There are sound legal, moral and economic reasons to prevent them from having accidents.

Safe working practice is an essential part of good management and good workmanship. It must be part of an ethos accepted by both management and workers. It has to be endorsed from the highest level of management and applied by even the most junior worker. For this to occur, a clear safety policy must be understood by every member of the workforce, and the organisation and resources must exist to enable the policy to be implemented. It is clearly pointless to dictate that personal protective equipment should be worn, and then fail to provide or maintain it. The safety policy must also apply the best available knowledge with regard to the subject.

Safety requires the ability to avoid both the unplanned and unpremeditated accident that could result in personal injury as well as the planned, premeditated assault. Safe working practice is a technique of anticipating and controlling events so that injuries do not occur. It requires knowledge, skills and appropriate attitudes to ensure that suitable control systems are in place.

Accidents do not always result in serious injury. Indeed, more often than not there is a 'lucky escape' that harms little more than pride and dignity. There are many instances where people put themselves at risk without realising it, and get away without any adverse consequences. These occasions should not be ignored, for they are 'critical incidents'. Luck is not always present – inevitably one day it will run out. The law of averages means that if a potentially hazardous situation is repeated often enough, a proportion of occasions will result in property damage, in a smaller number there will be minor injuries, and in a few cases there will be serious injury or death (Fig. 1.1).

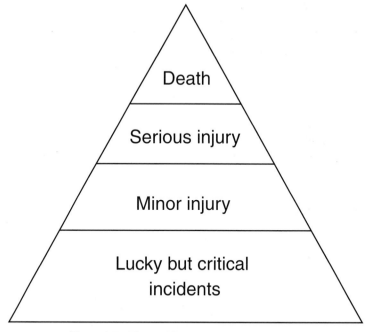

Figure 1.1 The accident consequences pyramid.

According to Bird and Loftus (fire service training leaflet, 1969), who have researched the character of accidents, there are five stages through which an accident evolves. These are as follows:

- a failure of organisation to prevent risk factors
- the presence of basic causes
- an unsafe way of handling the risks
- the incident
- the loss to health or property caused by it.

ORGANISATION

Organisation can prevent accidents by the co-ordinated application of four management principles (Box 1.1). The *Titanic* disaster is a clear example of the failure of the first three principles, and the debate continues about the quality of the accident investigation. The captain's desire for speed showed a serious lack of control. The fact that the radio operators ignored the ice warning and the watch had no binoculars showed poor monitoring, and the inadequate provision of lifeboats showed a lack of emergency planning.

Box 1.1   Management principles for accident prevention

Controls

The production of a safety policy for the situation provides objectives and standards of safety that should be communicated to all those involved.

Monitoring

Effective monitoring of the implementation of the safety policy ensures compliance. This identifies the need for further training, disciplinary procedures or further investment to provide continuing safety.

Emergency planning

Despite the best intentions accidents can, and will, happen. Emergency planning is a strategy that minimises the effects of an accident.

Accident investigation

This is the only way that experience can be gained from one accident to help prevent another.

BASIC CAUSES OF ACCIDENTS

The causes of accidents can be divided into three basic groups. There are the human factors that cause accidents; there are also environmental factors that influence the likelihood of accidents; and, finally, there are task-related influences on the development of accidents.

Human factors

Stress is possibly the greatest cause of accidents. When people have too much on their minds, they are unable to spend adequate time on any one problem. Consequences are not fully considered, mistakes occur, and safety factors are forgotten.

Personality is another major factor. Some personalities can cope with stress better than others; some personalities are more conscientious than others; and some can inspire the loyalty of their workforce more than others. Some individuals are better motivated than others to ensure standards are maintained.

Physique inevitably can affect a person's ability to perform a task, and a certain level of physical fitness must be expected from emergency personnel if they are not going to be a risk to both themselves and their colleagues.

Intelligence is essential when faced with new problems. At any emergency there is the need to be able to deduce the best approach to the problem lying ahead. Low intelligence means the ability of deduction cannot keep pace with the speed at which the incident is evolving.

Environmental factors

The environment in which we work has a major effect on the likelihood of accidents. Noise can prevent us from hearing approaching danger; poor lighting, rain or dust can prevent us from seeing it. The environment can be unstable, but this may not be apparent. Cold or excessive heat can distract and exhaust us. The vast majority of this book is devoted to explaining the risks of different environments and the techniques for safely overcoming them.

Task-related factors

These can be reduced by accurate assessment of risk, proper training to undertake the task in a safe manner and the provision of equipment that is appropriate, effective and ergonomically designed. Appropriate scheduling of work patterns, with adequate rest breaks and refreshment, can reduce fatigue. Above all, providing staff with the experience necessary for them to be able to undertake the job effectively influences the safety of the task undertaken.

UNSAFE HANDLING OF RISKS

Eighty-eight per cent of all accidents are caused by an unsafe act, or series of acts, that someone does. Good management and attention to the basic causes of accidents should leave a rescuer aware of both the risks and good working practice. Accidents can be minimised but will always occur because of the failings of human knowledge and behaviour. Always be aware that members of the public, and even your own colleagues, may fail to consider your safety. Make no assumptions and you will already be less likely to be an accident statistic.

KEY POINT

- Accidents can be minimised by good working practice.

Personal protective equipment

Personal protective equipment (PPE) is defined as being all equipment (including clothing affording protection against the weather) that is intended to be worn or held by a person at work and protects him or her against one or more risks to his or her health or safety.

The Personal Protective Equipment at Work Regulations 1992 (Department of Employment 1992) cover in some detail what is included under PPE and what is not. Clothing for adverse weather conditions, gloves, high-visibility waistcoats, eye protectors and breathing apparatus are among the items mentioned.

PPE cannot be regarded as a set of clothing that will protect the individual from all hazards. Indeed, what is protective in one environment will itself be a hazard in another. Some years ago several military recruits died of heat stroke when undertaking strenuous activity while dressed in wet suits on dry land; this illustrates the danger of assuming that PPE is always safe.

RISK ASSESSMENT

For PPE to be appropriate the hazards associated with an incident need to be recognised. This hazard recognition needs to be part of the perception of the rescuer, not merely that of a management safety officer. If the need for an item is not perceived then it may well be discarded, as most items of PPE have disadvantages associated with them. This hazard recognition introduces the need for a risk assessment. Over the centuries rescuers have been injured in many different ways. The question that has to be addressed is whether the cost of providing protection is justified by the risk. Introducing a new piece of safety equipment into a service is expensive, and will inevitably mean less money is available for patient care and salaries. Many paramedics may prefer a pay bonus to having to wear body armour, but attitudes would change rapidly if a stabbed paramedic's widow was told that the bonus had removed her right to compensation.

The problem is not only a question of the statistical risk, but also one of perceived risk. During the Second World War allied bomber pilots were told by plane designers that if they removed the back-up systems for controlling the aircraft it could fly higher and avoid much of the anti-aircraft fire. However, the crews preferred to fly planes that were at greater risk of taking them to their death because they feared the thought of losing control of their aircraft, even though many more planes were shot down than ever crashed from primary control system failure.

Having assessed the risk, an appraisal of the type of protection required needs to be made. PPE should only be considered when changes in working practice fail to contain the risk. The use of intravenous cannulae that automatically sheath the needle on withdrawal reduces the risk of needlestick injury at scene, and while not making the use of gloves redundant, they do increase safety by reducing the probability of the glove being the last defence.

SELECTION OF PPE

Once it has been decided that an item of PPE is required there is still the question of which style and which manufacturer. Chemical protection against splash contact to the level deemed appropriate by the Ambulance Services Association can be provided in the UK at about £200 per suit. This is substantially cheaper than the other alternative system at around £400 a suit. One of the ways this saving is made is by substituting a power-ventilated respirator hood with a simple respirator mask. Military personnel are familiar with this equipment and have trained extensively with it, but paramedics and immediate care doctors would have less extensive training and could well become more claustrophobic with masks than with ventilated hoods. A panicked removal of the mask would remove all the protection the suit offered, and so it is likely few ambulance services will adopt them.

PPE needs to fulfil the following functions:

1. It must protect the head (and brain within it) from injury.
2. It must protect the eyes from physical, chemical and biological risk.
3. It may need to protect the ears from acoustic trauma.
4. It may need to protect the body from fire, hypothermia, lacerations and chemicals.
5. It may need to protect the respiratory system from chemicals or dust, and may need to be able to supply clean air to breathe.

6. It must protect the hands from lacerations, needlestick injuries, and biological and chemical risks.
7. It must protect the feet from injury and exposure to chemicals, etc.
8. It may need to protect the person from physical injury because of falls or assaults.

There is a level of PPE that rescuers attending an out of doors rescue incident in the UK might be expected to have available. Higher levels of PPE could reasonably be expected to be provided by the fire and rescue services or alternatively by specialist rescue teams. It is essential that rescuers realise when their PPE is inappropriate for the risk.

Head protection

For the routine rescue scenario the building site bump hat does not offer adequate protection for the head. Several manufacturers produce appropriate helmets that meet national standards, the most commonly used being the Pacific or Cromwell helmet, with a visor that lifts above it. These have a tendency to catch on obstructions in confined spaces, and become covered in rain when raised in wet weather. The Gallet helmet is close fitting and has both integral visor and goggles, but some people find the adjustment to prevent the goggles and visor catching on the nose as they are brought down difficult to make. Gallet believe that by altering the padding within the helmet it can be made to fit everyone. A similar helmet, with integral visor but no goggles, is made by Cromwell. This meets the needs of the rescuer very well indeed, but the visor retreats into a cowl that distorts the smooth lines of the helmet, and it is possible that it could be an obstruction. Pacific also market a helmet with integral visor and streamlined holder for a high-intensity torch. While some of these torches are not marked as intrinsically safe, they are used by divers and are therefore totally sealed and safe in explosive atmospheres. Helmet visors alone are not adequate protection when cutting is in progress, and should always be used in conjunction with safety goggles or spectacles. Many people find that goggles are very prone to misting up when they are exerting themselves. This of course defeats the purpose of the PPE.

Ear defenders

Ear defenders need to be considered for noisy environments. Some safety officers may argue that they should be provided by the service that creates the noise, but PPE must be compatible, and some attention must be paid to ensuring that the ear defenders and the helmet can be worn together. Ear defenders are cumbersome to carry all the time and therefore are likely to be in your vehicle when you need them. Ear plugs on the other hand are small enough to slip into a pocket, and while they are not as robust, they have the advantage of economy and accessibility.

Protective clothing

The selection of clothing is a difficult issue. Unlike the firefighter, paramedics and doctors usually work in heated and protected environments. The protective quality of the firefighter's uniform would be inappropriate and uncomfortable in these situations. However, recent tests have revealed that the usual materials employed in paramedic green overalls are more flammable than paper! The Gemma suit made famous in HEMS (Helicopter Emergency Medical Services) videos is excellent but is also hot and heavy to wear. BASICS (British Association for Immediate Care) has recently produced a fireproof overall and this is probably a reasonable compromise between comfort, cost and safety.

Gloves

Medical staff should wear latex gloves to avoid blood pathogen inoculation, but such gloves are inadequate in the presence of glass fragments and torn metal. Barbour make 'thorn-proof' gloves that are resistant to this type of damage and have removable tips to thumb, index and middle fingers, allowing considerable sensitivity of touch. The standard latex glove should be worn underneath to provide a barrier to body fluid contact. Barbour gloves do not match the resilience of firefighter's gloves.

Boots

Wellington boots are often provided as they have the advantage of fitting a multitude of potential wearers. The problem with Wellington boots, however, is the poor grip that occurs between foot and ground, either because of slippage of the foot in the boot, or of the boot on the ground. Merely having steel toe caps and steel insoles is not enough to ensure that boots conform to the recommended safety requirements. They may have severe limitations in resistance to chemicals. Many fire services have moved towards the use of a specially designed leather firefighter boot. These are remarkably comfortable, meet all safety standards, and give excellent grip on the ground.

MANAGEMENT OF PPE

According to the Personal Protective Equipment at work Regulations, PPE is not deemed to be suitable unless it is appropriate for the risk involved, takes into account ergonomic needs and the health of the wearer, fits correctly, complies with legislation, and increases safety without increasing the overall risk. The Guidance Notes for these regulations suggest that PPE should only be used when 'Safe Place' and 'Safe Practice' principles fail to prevent risk. PPE should be supplied on an individual basis, and no charge may be made by the employer for it.

Where more than one item of PPE is worn, all items must be compatible to ensure they give adequate protection when worn together. Thus it should be possible to wear ear defenders and a helmet with visor when required.

It is the duty of the employer to ensure that any PPE provided by them to their employees is maintained in an efficient state, in good working order and is cleaned or replaced as soon as possible. The equipment must have been assessed as suitable for the task involved. The employer is responsible for the proper training of the employee in the correct use of the equipment. Decisions with regard to PPE must be regularly reviewed by the employer to ensure that the policies and equipment continue to be valid and effective. The employer is responsible for providing appropriate accommodation for PPE when it is not being used; this should protect the PPE from contamination, loss or damage. The employer is also responsible for ensuring that the employee understands the risks that the equipment will avoid or limit, the manner in which it is to be used, and the manner in which its efficiency is to be maintained. Depending on the complexity of the equipment, retraining may be considered essential.

Employees must use PPE provided in the manner in which they were instructed. The PPE must be stored in the accommodation provided for it when it is not in use. Employees are responsible for reporting to the employer any defect in the equipment.

KEY POINTS

- PPE must not be considered to provide absolute security.
- PPE should be used when working practice fails to eliminate the risk.

Self-test questions for Chapters 1 & 2

1. What are the five stages of an accident?

2. What is a 'critical incident'?

3. State four management principles for safe working practice.

4. What are the three basic causes of accidents?

5. List four items of personal protective equipment that should be worn when at a road traffic accident requiring casualty extrication techniques.

Answers on p. 205.

3

Going mobile to scene

It is not the remit of this manual to be a comprehensive guide to safe driving practice or the correct approach to an incident. This is such an extensive subject that it is a full course in its own right. It is essential, however, that you 'drive to arrive', and don't let your attention become fogged by the 'red mist' that comes when you are swept into the drama of unfolding events.

VEHICLE PREPARATION

Ambulance services should have a fleet of vehicles that are not only correctly marked up with high-visibility stripes and warning signs, but also fitted with blue lights and horns. The vehicles should be regularly maintained to ensure their roadworthiness for emergency response considerations. If you are an immediate care doctor or an ambulance officer who responds in your own car, it is essential that the mechanics who work on your car realise that you do response driving in it. Emergency vehicles also need regular cleaning to ensure good all round visibility, clean lights and effective reflective markings.

The next issue is that of warning beacons. The Road Vehicles Lighting Regulations (Department of Transport 1989) state that an emergency vehicle includes 'a vehicle used for fire brigade, ambulance or police purposes'. Therefore any immediate care doctor's car attending an incident at the request of the ambulance service is deemed to be an emergency vehicle. Regulation 11 (paragraph 2) states that no vehicle shall be fitted with a lamp that is capable of showing any light to the rear, other than a red light, except:

(o) Blue light from a warning beacon or rear special warning light fitted to an emergency vehicle.

(p)   Green light from a warning beacon fitted to a vehicle used by a medical practitioner registered by the General Medical Council (whether full, limited or provisional registration).

Regulation 13 states that no vehicle shall be fitted with a lamp that automatically emits a flashing light (unless):

(l)   it is a headlamp fitted to an emergency vehicle.

This means that to use flashing headlights you must be an emergency vehicle.

Regulation 27 also states that blue warning beacons and lamps shall only be used at the scene of an emergency or when it is necessary or desirable either to indicate to persons using the road the urgency of the purpose for which the vehicle is being used, or to warn persons of the presence of the vehicle or a hazard on the road. A green warning beacon shall only be used by a medical practitioner for the purposes of an emergency.

Exemption from various other parts of the Road Traffic Act 1989 (Department of Transport 1989) only applies to emergency vehicles. It would appear therefore that immediate care doctors attending an incident at the request of the ambulance service have the option of using blue or green lights, but if they use green lights they have no other privileges with regard to flashing headlights, two-tone horns, or speed limits. If they attend an incident as a general practitioner then blue lights cannot be used and the vehicle is not an emergency vehicle within the law.

The question remains as to whether green lights or blue lights are the safer ones to use when responding to an incident. There are proponents of both views. The blue light supporters argue that the average road user still does not understand what they should do when they see a vehicle with a green light approaching, and there are so many cars working for doctors' co-operatives that use lights when travelling within Road Traffic regulations that the intentions of the vehicle are more confused. The green light supporters argue that cars with blue lights are usually thought to be police cars and some members of the public will deliberately try to impede the progress of a police car, whereas if they see the vehicle is a medical one they would give way. Having driven with both types, I am now firmly in the blue light camp.

Magnetically mounted beacons, and to a lesser degree magnetically mounted reflective markings, can be a hazard both to your vehicle and to other road users if they detach at speed. Most manufacturers have a disclaimer against this. Some manufacturers recommend having a knot in the cable just within the door so if the light does detach it will not come completely adrift of the car. Certainly the wire inside the car should be routed to avoid the deployment path of any airbag.

GOING MOBILE

The rule of immediate care is 'always keep your tank full, and your bladder empty!' And broadly speaking this is the basis of safe mobilisation. The car should be ready to be driven before you set off. Ideally the car will have been garaged so there is no winter frost to remove from the windows, and no risk of vandalism.

If you have been caught with a full bladder it is logical to empty it before setting off. Similarly if you are about to eat, then a glass of milk and a biscuit can prevent both hunger pangs and the low-grade hypoglycaemia that can interfere with rapid decision making. Dress appropriately for the weather, preferably putting your overall on before setting off. The pressure to get started as soon as you arrive at the scene may encourage you to leave this component of personal protective equipment in the back of the car, risking at best a ruined suit and at worst your life. It is probably wise to leave the high-visibility jacket off until you arrive, however. The jacket restricts free movement within the car, and can cause you to become too hot, but most importantly it can prevent the lap strap of the seat belt from sitting snugly on the iliac crests. If you slide under the lap strap (a process called submarining), then you risk ruptured abdominal viscera, a ruptured diaphragm, and bilateral knee and popliteal artery injuries. The seat belt needs to be pulled firmly across the body and all slack taken up by the reel.

If the car is your own, and you were the last driver, then there should be little required in the adjustment and testing of controls before setting off. If you are the driver of a hospital response car or a car used by several family members, then you should follow a starting drill. The example given in Box 3.1 is from the Lancashire Constabulary Driver Training Section.

If you are unsure as to the location of the incident, or the route, then you should do your map reading before you start off. The advantage of this is not only that you will travel more rapidly and avoid an embarrassing stop because you're lost, but you can also remind yourself of sharp bends and other road problems you will encounter. Never try to drive and read a map at the same time.

Box 3.1 Starting drill

Outside the vehicle check the exterior to ensure that all passenger doors, bonnet and boot are secure and that tyres and wheels are in order. After getting into the vehicle:

1. check that the handbrake is on
2. check the driver's door for security
3. adjust the driving seat
4. secure the seat belt
5. adjust the driving mirrors
6. test the brake pedal for pressure
7. depress the clutch
8. place the gear lever in the neutral position
9. start the engine with the clutch depressed
10. check instrument lights, exterior lights, wipers
11. select appropriate gear
12. check mirror and over shoulder
13. move off when safe.

EN ROUTE TO SCENE

Police officers are taught to drive to a system of car control, the purpose of which is to provide an approach to hazards that is safe, systematic, simple and applicable in all circumstances. It has been in use since 1936 and, although minor variations have been made to account for modern vehicles, road engineering and traffic conditions, it remains essentially unchanged. As any drive along the road progresses, various problems are encountered. All these hazards need to be negotiated in a systematic manner. The police driver's manual *Roadcraft* (Department of Transport 1990) explains the philosophy and should be on every emergency vehicle driver's bookshelf. Driving requires more than a knowledge of principles, however – it also requires you to learn skills. It is for this reason that a driving course is so important.

The speed at which you travel must be dictated by the road conditions, and never by the severity of the accident you are attending. Generally it is felt that to exceed the speed limit by more than 20 mph is difficult to justify, and at times the speed must be less. There is an objective definition of 'dangerous driving', and it is generally held that an emergency vehicle driver should have been made aware of safe driving practice. It is therefore easier for the police to prove dangerous driving because the driver has been taught to know better.

Immediate care doctors are often unsure about the use of two-tone and other horns. The use of horns at speed on a motorway is pointless as the sound cannot escape the bow wave of air compressed at the front of the car. They should also not be used at night when traffic is slight and the disturbance will outweigh any benefit. If stuck in single-lane traffic some way back from the front of the queue, then continued use of the horns may precipitate foolish actions by those in front. Horns should be controlled in such a manner that operating the switch can be done without having to look where your hand has to go. Modern horns tend to be used as a wail on straight stretches, changing to a yelp when approaching a road junction, but there is no fixed rule and there is no convincing evidence that the sounds carry better in either circumstance. Generally horns should be used well before approaching hazards. You do not want to be operating the siren at the same time as looking in your mirror and signalling. Look for signs that the driver you are approaching has noted your presence. The driver may be playing loud music or may be deaf, or may be day dreaming or even drunk. If you are not sure that the driver has realised you are there, then be prepared to take evasive action if you decide to commit yourself to passing. Do not operate the horns unnecessarily. Not only can you cause nuisance, you can also fail to hear radio messages that may be of importance.

ARRIVING SCENE

Particular care should be taken when approaching an incident. The cause of the accident may be ice or oil on the road; the accident location may be incorrect; and it may be closer than you think. There may have been another accident because of traffic braking, or due to 'swan-necking' motorists passing by. Look for the motorway matrix signs, but remember that if you are first there the signs may have been incorrectly set. If this is the case you should inform your control at once.

As soon as the accident is seen consider a radio message that you are 'arriving scene'. If there is an ambulance crew on site they may well hear the message and be ready for your arrival. As you get closer to the accident your concentration will be on many other factors, so it is better to call early than late. Slow your approach as this gives you more time to read what is happening. Casualties or debris may be in the roadway. You need to get close to the casualties but you want to park safely, where you won't cause an obstruction, and from where you can escape later. On motorways the police now try to limit the show of blue lights so that they do not flash to the front of the accident. This means a fair proportion of motorists on the opposite carriageway will never notice the accident and the risk of swan necking is reduced.

When manoeuvring towards the scene try to be aware of any tyre marks (which may just be in the dew) and any debris or deposits on the road. The police may well be faced with preparing evidence for three courts: the coroner's, the criminal and finally, often years later, the civil courts. If someone is permanently handicapped because of the actions of another driver, compensation can be important. Evidence can be lost through rescue services failing to appreciate what constitutes such evidence and the importance of preserving it. The stretching of a bulb filament can mean that the vehicle involved had its lights on; four small deposits of dirt in the road may indicate the point of the first impact; and the positions of items thrown from the vehicle give information about the speed. Talking to accident investigators can help both them and you, as you will appreciate mechanisms of injury better than ever.

PROTECTION OF THE SCENE

If the police are not in attendance, or if the incident is not protected, then vehicles should be parked to defend the scene and personnel should dismount from the safe side. Traditionally this has been achieved by parking the vehicle in the 'fend-off' position, but there is currently debate between services as to whether there are better alternatives. It is worth seeking the guidance of your service or local traffic police. No one should be allowed to work or step outside the protected area. Vehicles that are used as 'fend-off' appliances must have all warning lights on. Most vehicle batteries will not power warning lights for very long before they are flattened. The engine is best left running, this situation being an exception to the road traffic legislation.

4

An overview of incident management: road traffic accidents

GENERAL CONSIDERATIONS

In the UK the overall responsibility for any accident scene lies with the police, unless fire is actually present, when the responsibility rests with the fire brigade until that fire is out. At all incidents, however, the police will rely upon the advice of the fire service with regard to safety. The Fire Service Circular 13/83 (HM Fire Inspectorate/Home Office 1983) clearly defines the fire service as the principal rescue service.

This is only sensible, since the fire service has both the rescue tools and the personnel, as well as the absolute authority when it comes to the safety of the scene. Thus the police will provide an outer cordon, and within the inner cordon only fire and ambulance personnel will operate. Ambulance personnel and immediate care doctors do not have authority to overrule the fire officer present, merely being able to advise them of the consequences of any actions on a casualty.

The individual emergency services all have their own responsibilities and interests, and these can conflict with each other. It is only by mutual co-operation and understanding that the most effective management will occur. When casualties are seriously injured the medical services will be attempting to achieve the 'platinum 10 minutes' and certainly the 'golden hour'. Speed is not a good bedfellow with safety and the two will only co-exist with harmonious working practice. This can only be achieved by the individual services training together. This concept is known as the 'team approach'.

Roger Snook was a consultant in accident and emergency in the 1970s who had a special interest in road accidents. He taught firefighters for many years at the Fire Service College, Moreton-in-Marsh, Gloucestershire. It was he who proposed to certain instructors at the college that there was

17

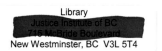

an alternative to the way that road traffic accidents (RTAs) were handled. Successive individuals, among them Len Wilson and Mick McCarthy, challenged the orthodox wisdom of the *Manual of Firemanship* (HM Fire Inspectorate/Home Office 1967–present), which said pre-planning was impossible for road accidents, and developed the concept of the 'team approach'. This is now recognised as the best way to manage the modern-day moving vehicle collision (MVC).

POLICE CONTROL AT INCIDENTS

It is essential at every accident site that operations are managed to ensure that any evidence available at the site that may assist the investigatory bodies later is left as undisturbed as possible. Therefore, from the outset, control of the incident is a priority, and an inner cordon should be established as soon as possible.

Inner cordon

The inner cordon is established around the immediate scene of events; it represents the area of actual work. To the police the inner cordon is the area that encompasses all significant evidence; to the fire service it is the area that encloses all hazards; and to the ambulance service it is the boundary within which all the casualties lie. Within this area the highest standards of safety must be observed at all times. Access is restricted to authorised personnel only. The fire service retains a responsibility for the safety of all personnel inside the inner cordon. They may need to provide special protection for non-fire service personnel who are not supplied with the normal fire service safety training and equipment. This might include providing them with safety equipment and clothing, informing them of their roles and the roles of others, and making them aware of what action to take when hearing the evacuation signal. However, the fire service would generally aim to exclude such untrained personnel from risk areas.

The size of the inner cordon will be determined by the event. Designation of the inner cordon might be physical, using barrier tape, lines or hose lines; or imaginary, using agreed physical markers such as streets and sentries. Control of access to an inner cordon is normally the responsibility of the police.

Outer cordon

The outer cordon is established to prevent access by the public into the area used by the emergency services for support activities. It is not considered a hazardous area. Rendezvous (RV) points will usually be located inside an outer cordon. This will reduce problems caused by the public, as the police will generally exclude them from this area. However, if the outer cordon is not large enough, then locating a suitable RV might be a problem.

Restricted area

A third cordon can be established at incidents to represent a very dangerous area within an inner cordon. There is no agreed terminology for this at present, although the term 'restricted area' is often used. An example might be an area of potential structural collapse, explosion or chemical leak.

PROTECTION OF RESCUERS

Personnel should wear protective clothing such as helmets, goggles, gloves and high-visibility fire-resistant clothing. The appointed safety officer should not allow any personnel inadequately clothed to enter the inner cordon. Personal protective equipment has been considered in Chapter 2.

During extended incidents, or incidents that are consecutive, the officers at the scene should consider the needs of the rescuers for rest breaks and refreshments. At the end of difficult incidents the need for personnel to recover must not be forgotten. There are now two recognised psychological conditions that result from dealing with emotionally charged situations. The better known is post-traumatic stress disorder, which is characterised by anxiety, withdrawal and a proneness to physical illness. It has been held that counselling is the best way of avoiding this condition, but recent studies have questioned this view. The second condition is persistent duress stress disorder, although this is less well recognised. The emergency responder may well be able to cope with the pressure of work for many years, but then his wife becomes ill, his daughter's marriage is going through a difficult time, the clutch on his car needs replacing, and he attends an accident where the child killed looked just like his granddaughter. The accident is no worse than others he has attended in the past, but it is the straw that breaks the camel's back. Personnel officers need to be sensitive to the needs of the 'front-line' troops if the incidence of these conditions is to be minimised.

STAGES OF A RESCUE

In all crashes the rescue proceeds through the same stages.

1. Establishing scene safety and making contact with the casualty to ensure airway control and protection of the cervical spine.
2. Stablisation of the vehicle and glass management.

3. Gaining entry to the vehicle and continuing stabilisation of the casualty.
4. Creating space to provide casualty extrication.
5. Evacuation of the casualty to hospital.

Therefore on arrival at an accident scene, the crew of a fire appliance should aim to protect the scene with an accident sign (if not already deployed by the police), lay out a hose reel and one or two dry powder extinguishers, stabilise the vehicles, start to remove the glass from the vehicle, and gain early access to the casualty to provide airway control and cervical spine immobilisation. They would aim to complete this within 2 minutes. They will then start to lay out an equipment dump on a salvage sheet, and a similar sheet may be offered for medical and ambulance equipment.

During this time the officer in charge will be assessing the scene so that when the cutting equipment is ready he or she will be able to direct the crew to complete the necessary extrication procedure. The crew should be ready to make their first cut within 5 minutes of arrival. Paramedics and immediate care doctors arriving at the scene will be expected to initiate these phases if there is no fire service support at that stage, or, if they arrive after the fire service, to synchronise with these stages.

SCENE ASSESSMENT

The fire officer in charge at the scene has many factors to consider. Any decisions will be influenced by medical advice. The first decision is whether the rescue is a 'snatch rescue' or 'immediate release', a 5-minute rescue, or a 20-minute rescue. A 'snatch rescue' may be little more than a controlled pull from the wreckage, or it may be the use of hydraulic spreaders to give a crushed victim space to breathe, or it may even be using a hydraulic cutting tool to amputate a foot to release the casualty when fire cannot be controlled. The 'snatch rescue' is only rarely required. The '5-minute rescue' is used when the casualty needs to be extricated within the 'platinum 10 minutes' if the life is to be saved. The '20-minute rescue' applies to the stabilised casualty where technique and comfort are principal considerations.

Looking into the heart of the scene from the outside, the fire officer will look for issues of scene safety. He or she will seek to assess the numbers of casualties and their priorities for treatment, and will look for absolute constraints on the rescue. An absolute constraint to a rescue is one that cannot be overcome within the time available for a live rescue. A stone wall, a derailed locomotive and an incoming tide are all examples of absolute constraints. There is no option but to work around them. Sometimes, however, it is possible to confuse absolute constraints with relative constraints. A bus

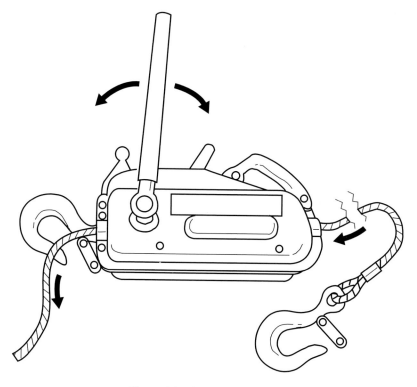

Figure 4.1   A 'Tirfor' hand winch.

that has fallen onto a car may appear to be an absolute constraint, but a Tirfor hand winch, set up by a firefighter with a knowledge of levers and winches, could right the bus in 15 minutes (Fig. 4.1).

The fire officer will also consider the evacuation route. If this is by ambulance, the fire officer will consider whether it is on the correct side of the accident site to enable its easy journey to the most appropriate hospital. If an air ambulance is to be used, where will it land? Do gates need to be opened, roads closed, ditches bridged? The fire officer will also consider the extrication path. How will the casualty come out of the vehicle? Are there hoses as trip hazards, or embankments that have to be climbed? Generally the extrication path should have been constructed before the casualty is disentrapped. Medical procedures such as ketamine anaesthesia may be needed for disentrapment, and the situation of the casualty who becomes unstable following the procedure, and yet cannot be extricated from the vehicle, needs to be avoided at all costs.

For all these decisions the fire officer will want to take advice from the attending paramedics or doctors. The fire officer will also need to look out from the inside. In other words, the fire officer will look for lack of airway control, asphyxiation, impalement, entanglement, entrapment and possible tamponade of abdominal haemorrhage by a steering wheel. The seat will be examined – does it recline, does it slide, is it powered? The fire officer will also look for undeployed airbags. These factors are considered in more detail in the chapters that follow to enable you to make a reasoned contribution to the fire officer's decision.

KEY POINTS

- Remember the 1–2–3 of safety:

  Personal safety – scene safety – casualty safety
- The police are in overall command.
- The fire officer has charge of the inner cordon until the scene is made safe.

5

Establishment of vehicle safety: road traffic accidents

The hazards that face a rescuer approaching a road traffic accident are numerous. Even if the site is protected from entry of further vehicles and the rescuer wears protective clothing, crashed motor vehicles pose numerous dangers. The first issues that need to be addressed are those of stability, chemical hazards and fire, as these need to be considered before any attempt to enter the vehicle is made. Some of the other major issues will also be considered in this chapter.

STABILITY

Stability of the vehicle needs to be achieved for three reasons. If a rescuer or rescuers enter a vehicle that is unstable, it may suddenly move, causing death or injury to both occupants and rescuers. As rescuers enter and leave a vehicle that is unstable the car can rock, thus exacerbating the injuries of the casualties as well as potentially causing sparks, etc. Finally, as the vehicle is cut apart the structural integrity may be destroyed, causing the vehicle to collapse suddenly. Therefore no attempt should be made to work on or enter any vehicle until full stabilisation of the vehicle has been carried out.

The fire service will commonly use step blocks adjacent to the wheels of the car to stabilise it (Fig. 5.1). These blocks are made out of reconstituted old car tyres, and are excellent for the task. They may be used in a variety of configurations, but the vehicle should not be rocked to put them in place, nor should they be kicked in place. The correct technique is to fit the step block as far under the sill as possible, and then push it firmly in place by tapping a wedge under it. The disadvantage of these step blocks is that they are black, and are therefore trip hazards, particularly at night. If knocked by a rescuer the blocks should immediately be

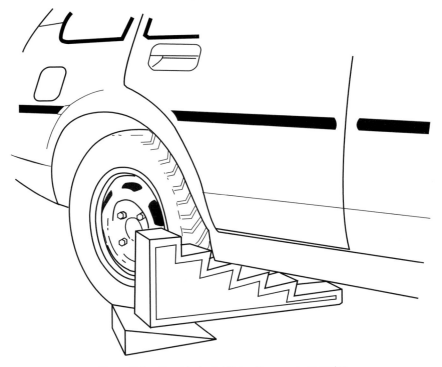

Figure 5.1 Step block stabilising the rear suspension.

repositioned so that they continue to perform their function. As the weight of the vehicle is reduced by removing its components the car may rise on its suspension, so stabilisation is a dynamic process and requires repeated checking (see Fig. 5.2). Stability may also be achieved by using ratchet straps, a Tirfor winch, ropes, etc. The sections of a triple extension ladder (Triple X) can be used to stabilise a car on its side by wedging the upper end of the ladder under the upper wheel and tying the bottom rung of the ladder to the bottom wheel with a line or the use of ratchet straps.

In multiple vehicle accidents it is not uncommon for a following vehicle to brake sharply, throwing the front of the vehicle down and low enough to under-run the car in front. The vehicles end up on top of each other, and stability is best achieved by strapping the vehicles together. This particular configuration of vehicles is a very great fire risk, as fuel from a ruptured fuel tank will spill directly onto the electrics below.

After stabilisation has been completed personnel should enter the vehicle as soon as practical to give moral and physical support to the casualty.

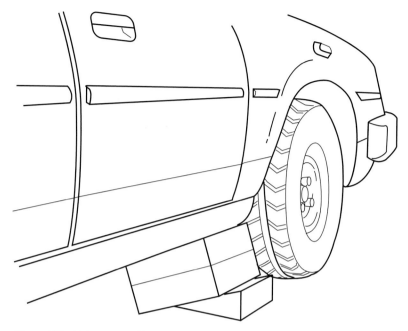

Figure 5.2   Using square blocks and a wedge for stabilising the front suspension.

RISK OF FIRE

Vehicle electrical system

It used to be taught that the power to the vehicle should be shut down because live wires act as a potential fire risk, but this may not always be the best course of action. If there is continued power to airbags they can deploy without warning, but airbags have a capacitor that can hold enough charge to trigger the bag for some minutes. Power to the fuel pump can cause continuing fuel leaks, while power to electric seat controls means they can be accidentally activated and cause further injury. However, use of the power seat adjustment can ease extrication if used correctly. The use of the electric windows may be the best way to gain access to the casualty as well as provide controlled management of the glass. Disconnecting the battery can also destroy valuable accident data in the on-board control modules.

Disconnecting the power is therefore no longer an automatic action but one that must be taken after a careful assessment of the incident. If the decision is taken to disconnect the battery, this should not be done by using bolt croppers on the cable, but if possible the battery should be disconnected by removing the **negative** lead. It is certainly wise to turn off the ignition as soon as possible, but **do not turn off the ignition without selecting**

neutral. Accidentally turning the starter motor with the vehicle in gear may injure the casualty further.

Fuel

Contrary to the image portrayed on films, cars infrequently burst into flames when they crash. Petrol from a ruptured fuel line does not ignite when it comes into contact with the manifold, or even with a catalytic converter. Sparks from a faulty high-tension (HT) lead or from short circuits occurring during vehicle deformation can ignite petrol, and brake fluid will ignite on contact with the manifold. Diesel fuel is considerably less flammable than petrol, but liquefied petroleum gas (LPG) does have particular hazards. A spill of LPG looks like water but is substantially below the freezing point of water. It will freeze and destroy living tissue on contact as it evaporates. It is highly flammable, and when confined it is explosive when heated. The use of water on an LPG fire will cause the flames to intensify, as heat energy is extracted from the water. The fuel is now more common, particularly in taxis, and the fuel is usually stored in the rear of the vehicle. When vehicles using LPG are involved in rear-end collisions considerable caution needs to be exercised. Cars are currently coming onto the market with dual energy systems, and some of these operate with electrical systems that generate over 200 volts. Cars are now being designed that will be fuelled by liquid hydrogen. These developments may create problems for rescuers that have yet to be fully evaluated.

Frequently the first bystanders to see an accident will report fire. This may be due to steam from a ruptured radiator, but this is white rather than the black of genuine smoke and there is no paint discoloration. Another phenomenon frequently confused with fire is the bicarbonate of soda, corn starch or talcum powder that is packed with the airbag to stop it sticking.

Prevention is better than cure, and turning off the ignition must never be omitted. Be very conscious of the use of high-flow oxygen in confined spaces. Approximately 3 gallons of pure oxygen is added to the atmosphere in the car every minute by this procedure. Within a few minutes the oxygen level in a closed car may be as high as 50%. This is a potent encouragement to combustion.

If fire starts while casualties are still in the car the situation may still be salvageable when the fire service are deployed. In their absence fire extinguishers will have only a limited effect. Bromochlorodifluoromethane (BCF) causes toxic fumes when it encounters fire and the only possibility of casualty survival is if a snatch rescue can be effected. In these circumstances there can be little attention afforded to the cervical spine and considerably more must be given to the rescuers' own safety.

On the arrival of the fire service the risks of fire and their management will of course become their responsibility. However, if you attend an incident before the fire service arrives, the deployment of bystanders to keep the area clear of unnecessary spectators, the prevention of smoking near the vehicles, the isolation of the vehicles' electrics, and the ready access to whatever fire extinguishers are available should all be considered.

GLASS MANAGEMENT

The most common cause of cuts at RTAs is broken glass. Procedures designed to reduce this are collectively known as 'glass management'.

At present all passenger windows fitted to cars are of the toughened type. It is, however, the intention of motor vehicle manufacturers to look at the possible fitment of laminated glass to all windows. There are two reasons for this: first, to reduce car theft from broken passenger windows; and second, to reduce injuries should the occupant's arm, leg or head fall from within the vehicle. This may also reduce the number of persons being thrown from the vehicle. A person thrown from a vehicle has a six-fold greater risk of death than a person who remains in the vehicle

There are a variety of devices for breaking toughened glass. A spring-loaded metal punch is the usual device used by car thieves, but these can become rusty and unpredictable as time goes on. The 'Life hammer' (Fig. 5.3) is an alternative and very effective tool, as is a new device on the

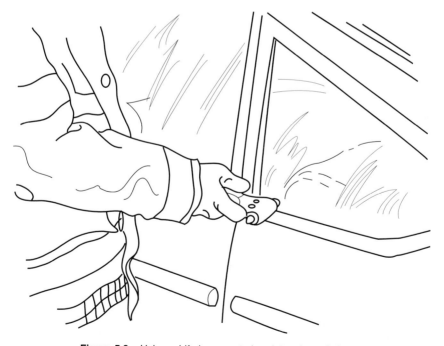

Figure 5.3   Using a Life hammer to break toughened glass.

market that uses the kinetic energy of a spring to give a controlled impact to the window. The corner of the window should be struck, close to the gasket. Gain access by breaking the rear quarter light rather than by spraying glass on the driver from the driver's side window. Ideally the glass is broken, and then the minimum amount gently pushed out to allow a gloved hand to release a door lock, etc., rather than pushing the whole of the window in.

Before a door is forced it is preferable to wind the window into the door so that only a centimetre shows, cover it with a sheet and then break the glass so it falls harmlessly into the door cavity. If the glass is merely wound into the door the stresses of cutting manoeuvres will almost certainly break the glass, which will then spray out of the gap and into the air.

Windscreen glass in older cars can also be removed in one piece by cutting the rubber gasket that holds the glass to give a strip to pull around the window, thus releasing it. Initially the blade of a stout knife should be inserted between the glass and the gasket and, using a cutting action, the central rubber core is cut through along a 9–10 inch (~25 cm) section, (Fig. 5.4), allowing a loop of upper gasket to be lifted from the screen. This is then cut halfway along the loop to give two handles. Grasp a handle of gasket with one hand and, using the other gloved hand in a sweeping action, the upper part of the gasket is separated from the lower (Fig. 5.5).

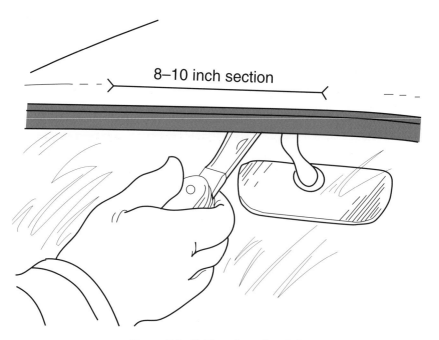

8–10 inch section

Figure 5.4 Cutting a loop of gasket.

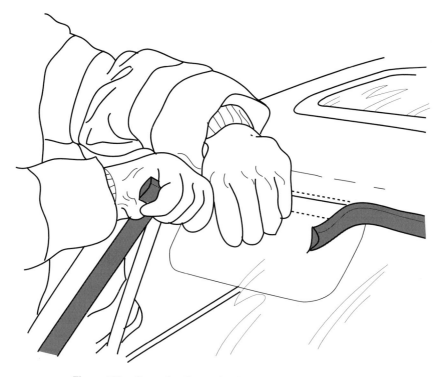

Figure 5.5 Sweeping the gasket from around the windscreen.

The glass has usually bonded onto the lower part of the gasket but will separate easily using the knife. The rear screen can be removed in the same way, but don't forget to disconnect the rear screen heater cables from their clips before pulling the screen away.

Laminated glass presents serious problems if glued in place. Bonding cutters such as the Kent tool work well with undamaged A posts and new cars where the bond has not hardened (Fig. 5.6). Older cars and those with distorted A posts need other approaches. One method that has been tried is to cut a 4 inch (10 cm) section out of the A post using the dedicated cutters and then use the dedicated spreaders to force the ends apart. The screen tears from its bed. An alternative is to use the saws now carried on pumps. But this is slow and produces many glass shards that could be inhaled or enter the eyes. Another option is the use of the 'Hooligan tool' (Fig. 5.7). This looks like a cross between a heavy-weight ice axe and a tin opener. There is no finesse in its use, which is in the manner of a tin opener (Fig. 5.8). Glass fragments are widespread. Self-adhesive polythene sheeting and water sprays have all been tried, but currently if glass has to be broken the casualty and any rescuer nearby should be protected with both hard protection and soft protection. The most common hard protection is a tear-drop

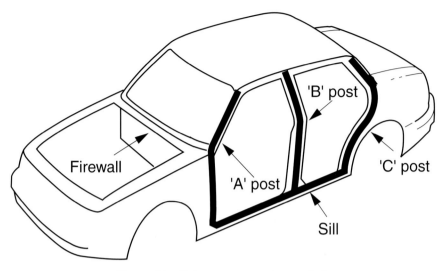

Figure 5.6 Major components of a car shell.

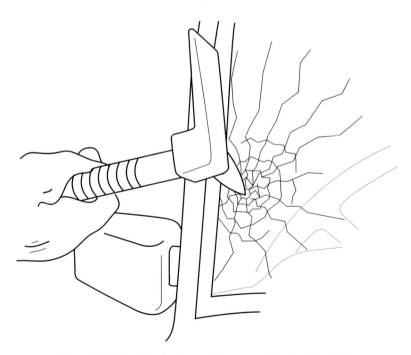

Figure 5.7 Breaking the laminated screen with a Hooligan tool.

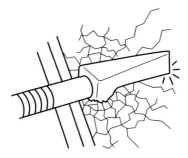

Figure 5.8   Using the Hooligan tool to cut the screen.

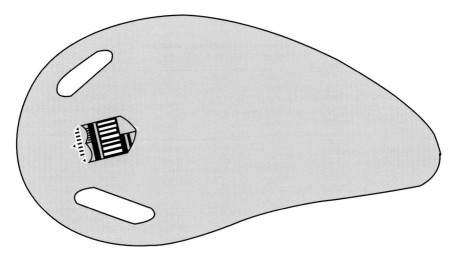

Figure 5.9   A 'tear drop' used for hard protection.

shaped perspex sheet that will deflect any projectile (Fig. 5.9). Soft protection has traditionally been a salvage sheet, but these are also used to cover
dead bodies and the claustrophobia induced while under one is not helpful
to the casualty. It is better to use the type of sheeting found on scaffolding,
which is tough but translucent. If glass is removed intact, then it should be
put outside the 2 metre zone or under the car so it can't become a toboggan.

   Always remember to protect the casualties' eyes when cutting. They
have a right to the same health and safety considerations as the rescuers.

KEY POINT

- Remember to consider stability, fire and glass management.

6

Extrication of casualties: road traffic accidents

TWO-METRE RULE

The use of hydraulic cutting equipment has revolutionised rescue techniques, but it introduces its own hazards and problems to the accident scene. Because of the tempo that needs to be achieved for the 'platinum 10' to be achieved, non-firefighters need to be aware of the actions of the tool operators to minimise risk of accidents. There are three key phrases that ambulance and medical personnel may need to use during the rescue: **Shut down**, **Hands off** and **Stand clear** (Box 6.1).

When using hydraulic cutting equipment at an incident the fire service try to keep all unnecessary equipment and personnel 2 metres away from the incident. This should also apply to ambulance crew and medical kit, as the intention is to remove trip hazards and allow room for when the casualty is removed from the vehicle. Fire crew rarely think to offer a salvage

---

Box 6.1 Key phrases for use during rescue

Shut down   This means the sources of noise need to be turned off, usually to allow an assessment of breathing with a stethoscope.

Hands off   This requires all rescue activity on the vehicle to cease in order to prevent any jarring movements that could foil a medical procedure such as cannulation.

Stand clear   This is to provide space for a particular manoeuvre.

---

sheet to protect medical equipment from the elements, but will happily do so if asked. Doors and other parts cut from the vehicle will be removed from the working area.

The power unit should also be kept as far away as possible to minimise the impact of noise or exhaust fumes, but it must be positioned so that the tools can be used to either side of the vehicle. Ideally the power unit will be placed to the rear or front of the vehicle, whichever takes fumes and noise away from the casualty.

The choice of equipment to be used will obviously depend on the type of incident and damage to the vehicle, and what rescue techniques will be employed to extricate the casualty. An understanding of the power of hydraulic equipment is important. There are several manufacturers of equipment and different fire services carry different brands. Most manufacturers make several grades of equipment. Fire services usually try to ensure that a 'first-strike' general purpose tool is widely available with heavier, more specialised equipment being restricted to incident support units or rescue units. The general purpose tool is often called a 'Combi-tool' as it is used for both cutting and spreading. Heavier tools are specialised to just one of those functions. A variety of rams is also part of the equipment. The hydraulic compressor used with this equipment also comes in various forms. Usually there is a manually operated pump. This is appropriate for pedal cutters but is unrealistically slow for use with any other tool. A small pump is usually designed for use with the general purpose tool and is operated in much the same way as a lawn mower motor. Heavy-duty pumps can operate two devices simultaneously. The pumps can create pressures up to 720 bar and the load applied can be around 7 tons. Blade failure is rare, but I have seen it happen and now have learnt always to wear both safety glasses and a visor. If the tool operator does not keep the shears at 90° to the cut the blades can separate and break. As the tool operates parts of the vehicle may themselves become projectiles unless restrained and objects such as doors will fall to the ground on an unsuspecting foot unless supported. Skilled operators will never place themselves between the tool and the vehicle as the tool can twist and trap them. The paramedic who realises this will have moved to allow the tool operator in, and thus save time.

The hydraulic hoses themselves should not be trodden on, but stepped over. They are very resilient, but the pressures they withstand merit respect. Firefighters have suffered catastrophic oil injection injuries after previous misuse has damaged the hose. The tool should never be put down on the ground with the blades apart and **never** be picked up by the blades.

ENTRY TO THE VEHICLE

The mode of entry will be dictated by the damage to the vehicle and what injuries the occupants of the vehicle have received. For example, if the damage is slight, first check that doors are available for use as this will avoid any unnecessary damage and save time. If the door will not open when the handle is operated, one person should hold the handle in the open position while another levers the door open with a crowbar.

However, if the vehicle has been involved in a major collision and has sustained a rear and front-end shunt, all doors may be severely distorted. It may therefore be necessary to remove the doors using hydraulic cutting equipment. It should be noted that when removing the casualty the hole should be made to fit the casualty and not the casualty to fit the hole. The principle is to cut metal away from the casualty without causing further intrusion into the vehicle. Cutting rescue techniques are described in detail in the next section.

CUTTING RESCUE TECHNIQUES

There are a number of techniques that can be employed to gain entry and allow the casualty to be removed from the vehicle; these are described below.

Side entry

Door removal

To allow the doors to be removed, the operator of the cutting equipment must first gain access to the hinges, as this is the most suitable point for removing doors.

This may cause problems because the doors may be severely distorted with no room available to allow the tips of the equipment to be inserted between the bodywork or posts and the hinges. If there is no room available for the tips of the tool, several methods may be adopted to gain access.

The most commonly used method is to crush the wing of the vehicle using the spreaders, which will open the gap between the doors and the posts (Fig. 6.1). Another method is to place the tool in the window opening with the jaws facing downwards, either directly adjacent to the lock or to the door hinges. When the tool is closed the door will crush inwards and should produce a small gap between the doors and the front or rear wing. The tool is then used to force first the upper hinge and then the lower hinge of the door. The intention of this sequence is to help prevent the door moving in on the casualty as it is forced. Finally, the Nader bolt, which is the metal pin into which the lock connects, is cut or forced. The process of door removal should only take 4 minutes, but cars vary and some can prove very resilient. The presence of side impact bars should not impede removal of doors in this way. Increasingly, however, plastic and polycarbonate skins are used to cover the wings and doors. This material is compressed by the hydraulic tool until it suddenly splinters, causing a wide spray of sharp projectiles.

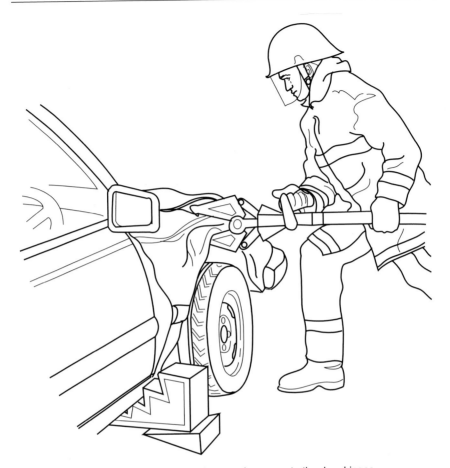

Figure 6.1   Crushing a wing to gain access to the door hinges.

Footwell clearance

By cutting through the A post at sill and dash level the metalwork of the internal wing that can conceal foot entrapment may be mobilised. The metal is either pushed out of the way with a power ram or pulled away using the leverage of spreaders. This process takes about 6 minutes (Fig. 6.2).

Fourth door creation

In the case of a three-door hatchback or estate the bodywork between the B and C posts can be removed (Fig. 6.3). This is achieved by cutting the B post high and low, and then cutting either vertically down in front of the C post (at the rear of the rear side window) or continuing the horizontal cut from the B post at sill level. Both cuts may be required. Leverage of the

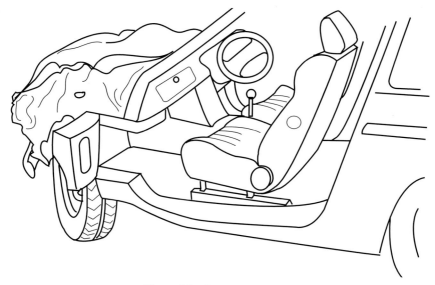

Figure 6.2   Footwell clearance.

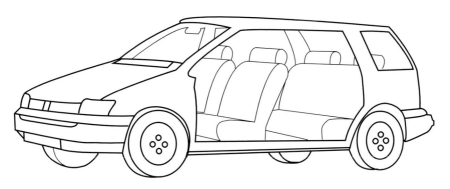

Figure 6.3   Fourth door creation.

isolated section of side wing will allow more room for manoeuvring the casualty, or reaching those in the rear seats.

The B post (American) rip

This procedure involves first forcing the Nader bolt of the rear door, then cutting the B post through the front and rear door window openings. A deep cut is made into the rear of the base of the B post at sill level and the spreaders used to force a tear through the rest of the post. The whole side of the car will then swing forwards on the front door hinges (Fig. 6.4). The

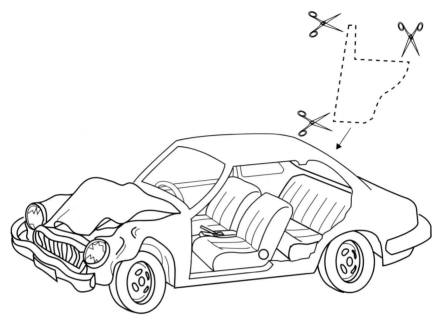

Figure 6.4 The B post rip.

technique takes about 12 minutes if all goes well, but rust in the sill of older cars means that the sill starts to crumble rather than the B post tear. The use of high-strength light alloy (HSLA) in modern cars at the foot of the B post can also complicate matters and skilled operators may take 20 minutes and more to complete the task.

The side fold down

The Nader bolt of the rear door is forced, the B post cut high, as in the previous procedure, and the door hinges at the front forced. A cut into the B post at sill level will then allow the side of the car to be folded down. This has the advantage of creating a stable working platform to stand on, but the side of a car also creates many trip hazards for the unwary.

Entry from the top

Roof removal

Most firefighters are conversant with removing the roof from a vehicle and the following points should be borne in mind when carrying out this task. Full roof removal is undertaken less frequently these days for various reasons. Carrying the roof away requires four firefighters and involves lifting an unsupported weight with sharp edges over the casualty and any rescuers within the car. A gust of wind or downdraught of a helicopter air ambulance would wrench it from the control of the crew. It also requires the laminated and bonded screen to be separated from the roof and it prevents its replacement if the weather conditions are bad. As a final complication, if the roof has been severely distorted and is in contact with the occupant's head, it will more than likely move towards the casualty, possibly causing further injury and pain.

It used to be taught that when cutting the posts they should be cut as low as possible to avoid injury. The increasing use of airbags located in the A posts and air curtain inflator cartridges in the C post, the presence of reinforced seat belt anchor points in the B post, and the use of HSLA and boron steel in roll-over protection systems (ROPS), all make it much more difficult to be didactic about the best level to cut.

It is good practice to cover the cut metal with salvage sheet or old hose to reduce the risk of injury. The tailgates on certain older estate cars have springs to assist the opening operation. When cut these can fly up with considerable speed and force, causing severe injury to personnel who may be unaware of the danger. This problem is not encountered on newer vehicles as they have hydraulic or gas struts, which may cause problems only when involved in fire.

Roof flap to the rear

When attempting to flap back the roof two deep incisions should be made on opposite sides of the vehicles to aid the flap back. The screen pillars are cut as low as possible (Fig. 6.5).

When the roof has been cut and flapped back it should be tied down to prevent it from being blown back by the wind or by the downdraught from an emergency vehicle or police helicopter that may have arrived on the scene.

If the roof has been severely distorted it may be impossible to flap it back without using some considerable brute force and movement to the vehicle, in which case it may be more prudent to remove the roof as a whole rather than risk causing movement to the vehicle. Remember that the seat belts must be cut before attempting to lift the roof off and away from the vehicle.

Forward roof flap

A very successful technique is to flap the roof forwards. This allows paramedics to work unhindered at the front of the vehicle while the C posts are cut. Either the B posts are also cut high and the roof flapped forwards on crushed A posts, or two cuts in the roof just behind the B posts will allow

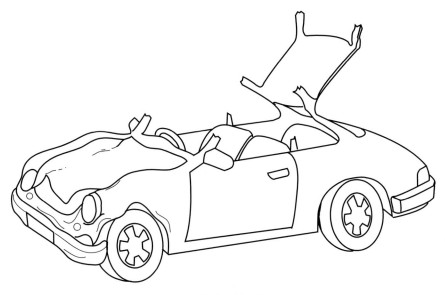

Figure 6.5 Roof flap to rear.

a crease to be created in the roof and just the rear part of the roof folded forwards (Fig. 6.6). When the front seats are reclined the access for a long
board is quite adequate. This is a rapid procedure even in inexperienced
hands, taking only about 4 minutes.

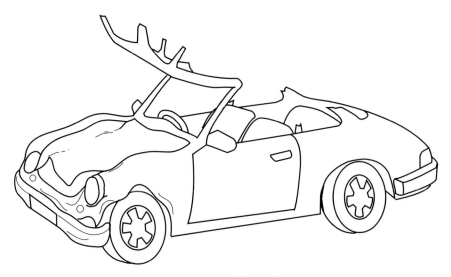

Figure 6.6 Roof flap to front.

Side roof flap

If the car is on its side it should of course be stabilised. Cutting the upper A, B and C posts and making relief cuts to weaken the bottom part of the roof will allow it to be folded down (Fig. 6.7). If the injured passenger is uppermost, two cuts may be made in the midline of the roof and half the roof folded away, leaving a ledge on which to rest the extrication board. This will not work in cars with a sunroof.

Entry from the rear

The removal of a tailgate from a hatchback is of course relatively straight-forward. But the boot lid, rear seats and parcel shelf of saloon cars may also be removed in about 10 minutes in older cars. Newer cars often have HSLA steel in the seat backs to help prevent injury from luggage in the rear crashing forwards. If the vehicle is distorted, then removal of the seat backs may be unexpectedly complicated.

The overturned car

The long board lower

This is a technique for where the casualty is suspended upside down from the seat by the seat belt. It requires the roof not to have been crushed. The

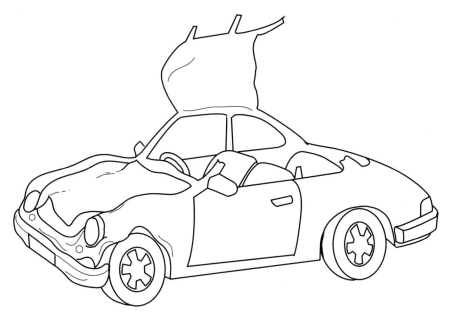

Figure 6.7 Side roof flap.

doors are forced and a ratchet strap, line or length of hose is used to take the weight of the casualty by passing across the width of the car and tensioning by two firefighters. The rear is also opened. A long board is passed along the roof of the car until it is below the casualty. The back of the seat is reclined, the seat belt cut, and the casualty lowered to lie prone on the board, which is then removed. This procedure can be completed in 10 minutes or less.

The inverted B post rip

In many ways this is an easier technique to perform than the classical version. It gives good and rapid access to the vehicle, and may then be further developed by conversion into an oyster (described below).

The rear oyster

This procedure is required when the roof is crushed to bonnet level. The C and B posts are cut on both sides and hydraulic rams are used on both sides to open the car like an oyster (Fig. 6.8). With two rams at their maximum extension there is a little loss of lateral stability, but two firefighters can provide all the lateral support required. This technique is quite quick if the vehicle is not too badly damaged, as in the training scenario. In real life, however, it can take a lot longer.

The side oyster

In this technique the A, B and C posts on one side of the vehicle are cut and a ram is used to open the vehicle along the side. This obviously requires the use of ratchet straps or Tirfor winch to maintain stability.

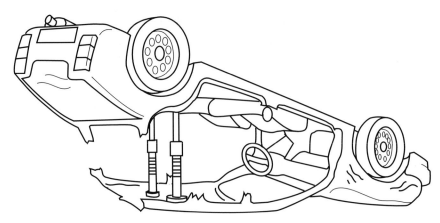

Figure 6.8   Rear oyster.

Lateral roof slide

This technique is appropriate if the casualty is lying on the roof and the weight of the car has collapsed onto it. It requires a crane or emergency tender with a hydraulic lifting hook. This is used to take the weight of the vehicle, with extra stability at the bonnet and boot provided by low-pressure airbags. The A, B and C posts are cut on both sides. The roof is then pulled from under the car to the side.

The floor pan cut

If the vehicle is upside down and access to door and rear is unavailable, then the only approach left is to cut access through the floor pan. Even with the new high-speed reciprocating saws this can take time, and the fact that the tool operator cannot see the casualty creates further hazards.

Disentrapment from frontal impact

Dash roll

If the vehicle has become involved in a head-on collision and the occupant has become trapped by the lower parts of the body, the method known as the dash roll may be used to free the occupant (Fig. 6.9). The first consideration must be to separate the upper part of the A post from its connection

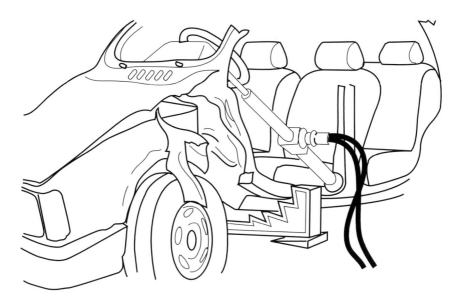

Figure 6.9   A dash roll.

via the roof with the B and C posts. This can be by a roof removal, a forward flap, or a rear flap

Next, two cuts will need to be made in the A posts directly beneath the hinges. It has been custom and practice to make these cuts in the sills. If these cuts are made in the sills, there is a possibility of the floor pan rising up and trapping the casualty's feet. Furthermore it is now common for fuel lines, hydraulics and electrical wiring looms to be located in the sill. It is therefore more practical to make the cuts into the A post directly beneath the hinges. Modern car design provides a further complication to this procedure in that newer cars often have substantial amounts of HSLA steel at the bottom of the A post to help prevent intrusion of the front wheel into the footwell. There may now also be a crosspiece of boron steel built into the dash structure, which would prevent a dash roll being completed with only one A post being cut through. The next step will be to place two rams, one in the passenger side and one in the driver's side. To ensure a smooth operation, the rams should be operated in unison.

Alternatively, one small ram can be placed with one end in the gear stick housing hole in the car floor and the other end under the dash and directly beneath the steering column; this can be very effective. If using one ram it must be remembered that the ram must touch the metal bulkhead. This is because on some vehicles there is some 300 mm of plastic between the dashboard and the metal. The blocks giving the vehicle its stability should be monitored at all times during the manoeuvre for any movement and readjusted if necessary.

A dash roll can even be undertaken without a ram, using ratchet straps running from chains attached to the rear half axles to chains across the dash.

Pedal repositioning or removal

In many cases pedals may not have to be removed and can be simply moved to the side by tying one end of a section of seat belt webbing to the pedal and the other to the edge of the door. Alternatively a pocket line can be used for this. By opening the door the pedal is levered outwards. Cutting the heel seam on the shoe or the laces may allow the foot to be freed.

If this method fails a mini-cutter may be used, but when using this piece of equipment it may twist with some severity, entrapping the casualty's feet or foot further.

Steering wheel relocation

This method of releasing the steering column away from the casualty uses the Combi-tool or dedicated spreaders in conjunction with chains supplied with the tools. The most rapid and effective alternative to releasing the pressure of a steering wheel on a casualty is to move the seat backwards, or to recline the seat. This should always be considered as a first option, and undertaken as soon as airway control and cervical spine immobilisation has been carried out. Furthermore the possibility that the compression of the steering wheel may be providing tamponade of abdominal haemorrhage must not be forgotten. The injudicious removal of the wheel before disentrapment is complete and the extrication route prepared could lead to the death of the casualty while still trapped upright.

Chains are wrapped around the steering wheel and attached to one blade of the tool with its jaws wide open. The other blade is attached by chains to the front axles of the car. Closing the jaws will pull the steering wheel away from the casualty. The casualty should be protected in case the chains should slip. A long board is ideal for this purpose. When carrying out the pull, rescuers should avoid standing in line with the chains.

The method should be backed up with the use of ratchet straps to prevent any backward movement of the steering column, should the chains slip or the spreaders require releasing to exert a further pull. When using this method the steering column has, on occasions, come adrift at the joint that joins the steering column to the rack and pinion steering box. This will then allow the steering column to move up and backwards towards the casualty with catastrophic consequences. This applies to front wheel drive vehicles and has been known to happen in the USA and occasionally in the UK. Because of this hazard the technique is now rarely used. It must therefore be remembered that if personnel are to attempt this manoeuvre, care must be taken to ensure that this will not occur. Furthermore this is a procedure that should **never** be used with an undeployed airbag.

Heavy goods vehicles (HGVs)

For larger vehicles the techniques used will depend on their construction. Most HGVs will have a more rigid chassis than a car and jacking will be possible in a variety of positions. However, some buses and coaches are constructed without a chassis and can only be lifted at certain points. Here, again, there are many types of lorries and quite a number of types of buses and coaches.

Many large vehicles today use air suspension units and personnel should be aware of the inherent dangers associated with these units. As the suspension system operates it is not uncommon for the wheels to turn a little. The air suspension unit will also tend to resist any lifting that is done on the chassis and it may be necessary to use blocks and straps to prevent any ride in the suspension unit. Lifting large vehicles without a crane is difficult. However, it is often necessary to lift only a small distance to release people trapped. It may be possible to achieve this by using the landing gear, or moving the lock-up wheel. Rescuers must not rely solely on the support of jacks, airbags or spreaders. Both during and after lifting they must place solid blocks securely to prevent the weight falling back on to a victim or rescuers because of an equipment failure. This method can also allow primary equipment to be withdrawn while large secondary, and more powerful, equipment is inserted to extend the lift or movement.

Rescue of drivers from HGV cabs has always presented many challenges, but modern vehicle design is making this particularly difficult. Lorry drivers are demanding the same levels of protection as afforded to car drivers, so airbags, air curtains and crush-resistant cabs are now being produced. Long-distance lorries are also being designed to cope with assault from hijackers, who, in some parts of the world, may be armed. Bullet-proof glass throughout the cab, with automatic locking and dead bolts on the doors, makes the cab almost as impregnable as a bank vault. Even with the heavy equipment carried on the incident support units or major incident support unit there may be a difficulty in cutting access. The structure of the A posts may be more complex than a simple box section, with several box sections within, and even a boron steel bar down the centre. Not only will the strongest rescue equipment be needed, but it will also need good tool technique and a knowledge of construction. This results in a greater entrapment time as specialist personnel and equipment are brought to the scene. Early attention needs to given to providing a working platform at a convenient height for the casualty care personnel. This may be provided by scaffolding, a flat bed lorry or even an extrication board used as a trestle, but before any structure is used a risk assessment needs to be made.

Recognised extrication techniques are described below.

Forward roof flap

In this technique the equivalent of the B and C posts are cut and the roof rammed forward (Fig. 6.10)

Half roof flap and dash roll

The A posts are cut, and after the roof has been nicked in front of the B posts a ram is used to lift the front of the roof. The A posts are then cut at sill level and a ram on each side used to perform the forward dash roll. This technique also works well with flat-nosed minibuses and delivery vans. Note that the emphasis is on using the ram to force the dash forward. It is tempting to use a winch to bring the dash forward, but many cabs tip forward for engine maintainance and are therefore only held down by catches. If these were to give way then the casualty would be propelled forward.

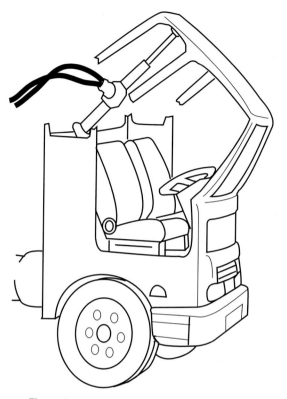

Figure 6.10   Forward roof flap on an HGV.

Three-quarter rear removal

This is a lengthy technique that requires the removal of the rear and side of the cab by use of the dedicated cutters, a reciprocating saw or even the carborundum cutting wheel (Fig. 6.11). It is worth remembering the rapid availability of heavy lifting equipment from private companies. The operators of this equipment are experts in their field and should be summoned early rather than as a last resort.

KEY POINTS

- There are standard techniques for extricating casualties from wrecked vehicles.

- A knowledge of these techniques improves liaison between emergency services.

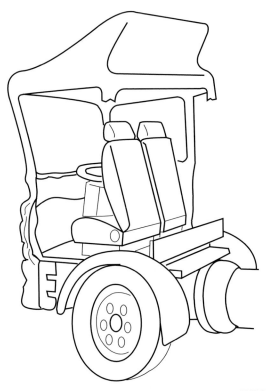

Figure 6.11 Three-quarters rear removal on an HGV.

HAZARDS POSED BY SUPPLEMENTARY RESTRAINT SYSTEMS

Airbags

On attending an RTA you should be aware that it is quite possible, because of the nature of the accident, that the airbag(s) fitted have not operated. To deploy an airbag fast enough to be effective impact detectors will detonate an explosive charge of sodium azide located in the steering wheel. This produces a massive release of nitrogen gas that forces the bag through a flap in the centre of the steering wheel. It inflates at 700 pounds per square inch until the large exhaust ports at the bottom of the bag are pulled from the housing as it reaches full inflation (700 p.s.i. is equivalent to ~4.8 MPa). At this point the nitrogen exhausts under pressure and at approximately 300°C, deflating the bag rapidly.

There are a series of issues regarding the arguments for airbags in the first place. Airbags were first used on some top-of-the-range American cars in the 1960s. These were highly effective systems that had mechanical systems to gauge both body weight and body position in relation to the airbag. They were, however, extremely expensive. The mass-produced American airbags had none of this sophistication and were high-volume bags because of the space within American cars.

From the date of their introduction to the beginning of 1998 there were 2.25 million driver airbag deployments and 344 000 passenger airbag deployments. They are generally accepted as having saved 2954 drivers and 494 passengers. As of 1998 there had been 113 confirmed deaths from airbags. Of these 15 were in rear-facing child seats and 51 were children, all of whom were incorrectly restrained. There were 42 driver fatalities, only 11 of whom were restrained, and five adult passengers died, only two of whom were restrained.

There is estimated to be a 31% car driver fatality reduction with the use of airbags and a 27% reduction in fatalities for car passengers where they are fitted. There is no doubt that airbags can save lives, and they are becoming much more widely fitted to cars, not only as steering wheel and dash-mounted bags, but also fitted in other locations.

An airbag is designed to deploy and deflate in about 120 milliseconds. This is faster than the blink of an eye. There is no possibility of a steering wheel airbag remaining deployed and obscuring vision, though the explosion (around 90 decibels) has been reported to have caused permanent hearing damage and can certainly stun a driver. The bag is packed in talc, corn starch or bicarbonate of soda to enable its smooth deployment. This can irritate the eyes and also give the appearance of smoke, suggesting the car is on fire.

Another problem is deployment of the bag during a high-speed shunt, such as colliding with a vehicle on an adjoining motorway lane. While with no deployment it may be possible to bring the car safely to a halt, if the bag deploys the shock to the driver would prevent any control being maintained. These, however, are issues for consensus between governments and manufacturers; the problems for rescue personnel are different.

The airbag's impact sensors will only deploy an airbag if there is a frontal impact within 20° of the midline on either side. The airbag would not necessarily deploy in the classic 'wrapped the car round a tree' type of side impact. The result is that rescuers are then faced with working only inches away from an armed Class 1 explosive that has a firing mechanism that can no longer be relied upon, having been involved in a serious impact.

The Dayton airbag incident in Ohio, USA, which was captured on video, demonstrates the dangers. If a paramedic or immediate care doctor were in the deployment path when a bag detonated as a result of fire service cutting or extrication manoeuvres, then he or she would not only be projected into the face of the casualty, but would also have his or her neck thrown against the B post of the vehicle with a 700 p.s.i. force.

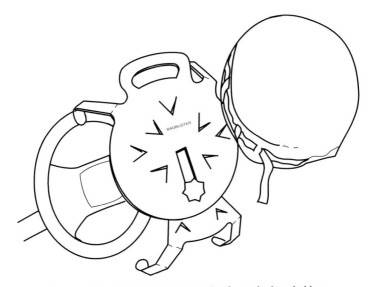

Figure 6.12   The 'Bag buster' device for undeployed airbags.

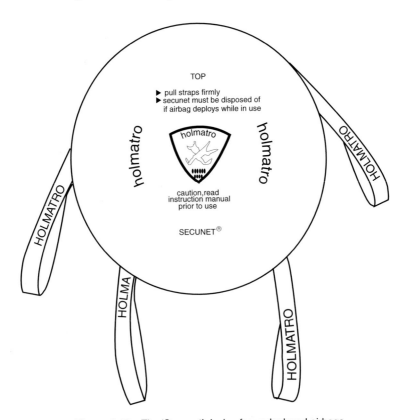

Figure 6.13   The 'Secunet' device for undeployed airbags.

Disconnection of the battery is not an answer as the mechanism has a capacitor that holds enough charge to detonate for up to 30 minutes. Certain extrication techniques such as steering wheel relocation will probably need to be abandoned, but the alternative of a 'dash roll' is still not without risk.

Within the bag itself particles of sodium azide will remain and with manipulation of the bag may fall into open wounds where they can be rapidly absorbed, causing a precipitous fall in blood pressure.

There are a variety of devices manufactured to provide protection to rescuers against accidental bag deployment (Figs 6.12, 6.13). Unfortunately, all of these are designed for the driver's airbag only. Airbags can be found in a variety of locations, and some top-of-the-range cars are now fitted with anywhere between 10 and 20 airbags. They can be located in the doors, side posts and seats (Fig. 6.14). Some are designed to inflate and deflate instantly, while others are designed to stay inflated until the car stops moving. However, the vast majority of modern cars have only a driver and front passenger airbag. If the driver is in a fit enough condition, he or she should be able to tell you if the vehicle has them installed.

Steering wheels containing airbags can sometimes be identified by the telltale moulded line that is the predetermined split line for the airbag breakthrough. Some cars have this score line on the inner face of the housing with no indication on the outer surface. Towards the bottom of the steering wheel

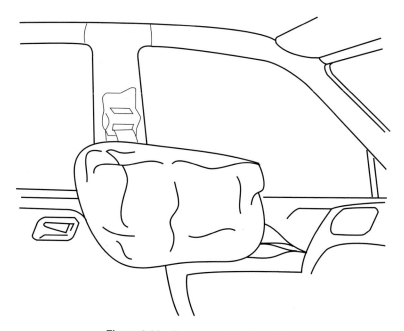

Figure 6.14 Passenger side door airbag.

may be moulded the word 'AIRBAG' or some other identification, e.g. 'SRS' (supplementary restraint system). In addition, a label may be visible on the rear edge of the driver's door just above the lock mechanism.

If there is an undeployed airbag, then you must try to avoid placing your body or objects against the airbag module, or in what would be the deployment path of the airbag. If possible, disconnect the battery by removing the **negative** lead. There is a theory – currently unproven – that once the battery terminals have been disconnected, touching them together will dump the charge from the capacitor and render all the supplementary restraint systems safe. As yet there is no-one who will take responsibility for the effectiveness of the method. Unfortunately an increasing number of vehicles carry a second battery, as the electrical power to supply all the luxury systems can drain the starter battery. In some cases this battery is to be found under the driver's seat! Cutting the spokes or rim of the steering wheel probably will not deploy the airbag and a dash roll should not deploy the airbag, even if the battery is connected.

Seat belt pretension systems

There are three impacts in every road traffic accident: the vehicle hits something; the person hits the inside of the vehicle; and the internal organs of the person hit the inside of the chest, skull or abdomen. The introduction of seat belts to restrain the movement of driver and passengers has undoubtedly been responsible for the saving of many lives, but the early models had intrinsic deficiencies. Seat belts have to stretch – if they did not, then they would not absorb any of the kinetic energy in the person and this would increase the severity of the second and third impacts. Seat belts stretch around 2 inches when subjected to a 30 mph impact. This stretching, combined with the fact that many people do not wear the belt as tight as they should, and the possible intrusion of the steering wheel into the car, mean that the traditional seat belt was unable to prevent the person from receiving facial injuries.

Systems that tighten the seat belt in the event of an impact are obviously advantageous but, like airbags, have to deploy at speed in the event of an accident. There are three main ways in which this is achieved. One system uses cables that tighten the seat belt as the engine is displaced into the passenger compartment. The other systems use spring-loaded buckles that retract, or explosives much like shot gun cartridges (Fig. 6.15). These may be located at the base of the B post adjacent to the seat belt reel, but are now more commonly to be found adjacent to the buckle. It is unlikely that they would fail to deploy, and then do so spontaneously later. Furthermore if they did so, apart from the noise and sudden tightening of the seat belt with possible injury to the casualty, the effects are minimal. The danger can be removed entirely by cutting the seat belt.

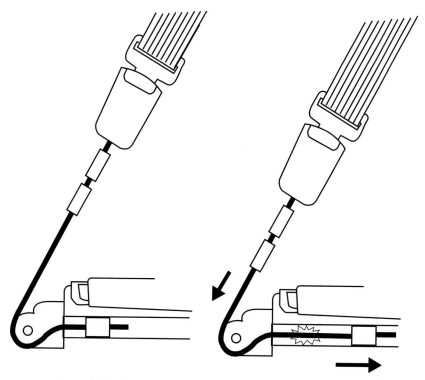

Figure 6.15   The mechanism of an explosive seat belt pretensioner.

Seat belts should always be cut because this serves two purposes. First, it is evidence for the police accident investigation team that the belt was on the person at the time of the crash (which may affect any compensation). Second, it stops any disreputable scrap dealer selling the belt since, as with crash helmets, once challenged they should be discarded.

The problem with fastening the occupant firmly into the seat is that this means the G-forces applied to the car are now also applied to the casualty. In excess of 4.5 G there is a serious risk of the third impact injuries being fatal. To try to minimise these injuries, such as aortic arch tears, liver, spleen and kidney injuries, the designers have produced G-force limiters. These are modifications to the seat belt drum assembly that allow a little more seat belt to be paid out if the G-force exceeds this load.

Automatic roll-over bars

Certain top-of-the-range convertible cars have automatic roll-over bar systems that deploy when the vehicle inclination exceeds anything between 20° and 50° or the vehicle acceleration is in excess of 0.4 G (Fig. 6.16). It

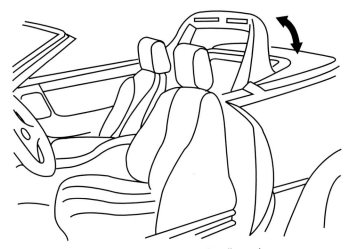

Figure 6.16 An automatic roll-over bar.

deploys as a result of tensioned springs in the housing of the roll-over bar. The undeployed roll-over bar can pose a hazard if the battery is not disconnected. Tools, rescue equipment and personnel should avoid the deployment pathway of the roll bar.

HAZARDS POSED BY BATTERY ACID, BRAKE FLUID AND OIL

These liquids are obviously an integral part of the car and can cause hazards in their own right. Oil will frequently leak from an engine at a road accident. This can be slippery enough, but when mixed with water or foam conditions can become extremely hazardous. The use of adsorbent materials can be very valuable.

Apart from the risk of fire from brake fluid, battery acid and brake fluid can cause problems in the overturned vehicle if they track into the passenger compartment. Battery acid is, of course, corrosive, as is the highly alkaline brake fluid.

KEY POINT

- Safety systems in vehicles can produce their own hazards.

Self-test questions for Chapters 3, 4, 5 & 6

1. What are the principal considerations that determine the actions of rescuers at a road traffic accident?

2. What controls do the police put in place at the accident scene?

3. Give two priorities in establishing vehicle safety after the scene itself has been protected.

4. What is understood by 'glass management'?

5. How do you remove a windscreen that is in a gasket?

6. Describe the main stages in a 'dash roll'.

7. When would you *not* use a steering wheel relocation procedure?

8. What should you check before you turn off the ignition?

9. How do you identify the presence of airbags?

10. Name five methods to extricate a casualty from an overturned car.

11. Why might an airbag fail to deploy?

Answers on p. 206.

Hazardous materials at scene

The number, quantity and variety of dangerous substances transported by road, rail or in the air is steadily increasing, and with it the risk of exposure following an accident. Safety in the industry is good. In 1995 the number of incidents involving chemicals on Britain's roads was only four per million tonnes. There are, however, some particularly toxic products being transported. There are even a few from which the fire service have no protection.

The possibility of dangerous substances being involved should always be borne in mind when assessing the scene of any moving vehicle accident. Hazardous substances may be:

- chemical
- radioactive (radiation hazard)
- biological.

Recently there has emerged the very real threat that an emission of one of these agents may not be due to accident or negligence, but to terrorist attack. The sarin gas attack on the Toyko subway system is a sinister development for rescue services. It is difficult enough to deal with a chemical incident when everybody is trying to help contain the situation. To deal with an unknown agent designed to cause injury and death without warning is a nightmare.

When dangerous substances are possibly present the management of the incident follows three basic principles: a careful **approach**, allowing a safe **identification** of the substance or substances, followed by an appropriate course of **action**.

APPROACH

The chemical industry is aware of the risks of incidents at processing and storage facilities. In conjunction with the local authority they will have produced plans to deal with any such incident. This will include defined approach routes that should be used. These are usually determined by wind direction and will therefore be dependent upon the day. If called to a chemical plant specifically check with your control whether a designated route has been stipulated, ensure you know what it is, and do not deviate from it.

In the absence of a designated route, the approach should be from upwind, in order to avoid any hazardous substances. Be aware that winds can veer suddenly, and so your approach should be with the wind full behind you, rather than to your side. Always be prepared to retreat if the wind changes direction. A stronger wind will produce a narrower footprint of contamination, but will spread the substance further (Fig. 7.1). The exact distance cannot be calculated without a knowledge of the size of particles released. Have regard to the fall of the land, as this can bring liquids towards you. Always try to approach from uphill. Be particularly cautious when approaching casualties who are collapsed or in severe distress. You may be overcome by an agent that has affected them.

Do not approach closer than is absolutely necessary – and is safe – to identify the substance involved. If the law is being adhered to then the substance should be correctly labelled; if this is in the UK Transport Hazard Information System (UKTHIS) format much information can rapidly be gained. Use of field glasses can be invaluable. As soon as any information that you are dealing with a chemical incident is available it is vital to inform your control. The sooner they are aware there is a chemical incident

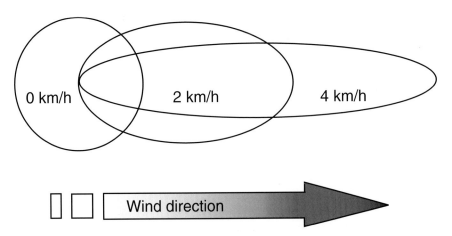

Figure 7.1 Effect of wind speed on the fall-out of an airborne chemical discharge plume.

the sooner specialist equipment can be mobilised and attending crews warned. There are many mnemonics to remind emergency personnel of the information to pass on, but in the absence of your service favourite the word ETHANE is valuable. The letters stand for:

E exact location
T type of incident
H hazards involved
A access route advised
N number of casualties
E emergency services at scene and required.

IDENTIFICATION OF HAZARDOUS MATERIALS

Materials may be in three physical forms:

- solid (powder, granules, crystals, pellets or molten)
- liquid
- gas.

Solids are generally found stored in drums of various sizes, but powdered chemicals can be transported in tankers. Liquids will be found in bottles, carbuoys, drums or tankers. Gases are found in cylinders. These may be of various sizes.

There is an International Classification System for Hazardous Materials. This is described in Box 7.1.

It will be apparent that identification of the suspect chemical is of paramount importance because without that information the correct method of handling it is unknown. To this end there are clear legal responsibilities with regard to the handling, labelling, transport, storage and use of hazardous materials.

Labelling of chemicals

The most commonly encountered method of labelling chemicals in the UK is the UKTHIS format. However, vehicles travelling on the mainland of Europe may use the ADR system. Both methods are described here.

United Kingdom transport hazard information system (UKTHIS)

The system provides rapid identification of individual dangerous chemicals, together with the hazard risk and method of dealing with them. All vehicles carrying prescribed dangerous substances in the UK are required to display warning labels on both sides and the rear (Fig. 7.2). In addition, companies are obliged by law to inform the drivers of tankers of the significance of the warning panels and the load carried.

Box 7.1 International Classification System for Hazardous Materials

Class 1

These materials are explosive. The class is divided into subgroups to denote the type of explosive hazard.

Division 1.1 Explosive with mass explosion hazard
1.2 Explosives with a projection hazard
1.3 Explosives with predominately a fire hazard
1.4 Explosives with no significant blast hazard
1.5 Very insensitive explosives
1.6 Extremely insensitive explosives

Class 2

The materials are all gases.

Division 2.1 Flammable gases
2.2 Non-flammable gases
2.3 Poison gases
2.4 Corrosive gases

Class 3

This class applies to flammable liquids.

Division 3.1 Flashpoint below −18°C
3.2 Flashpoint between −18°C and 23°C
3.3 Flashpoint between 23°C and 61°C

Class 4

These are flammable solids, spontaneously combustible materials and materials that are dangerous when wet.

Division 4.1 Flammable solids
4.2 Spontaneously combustible materials
4.3 Materials that are dangerous when wet

Class 5

These materials are oxidisers or organic peroxides. They may assist combustion or be destructive to cell structures.

Division 5.1 Oxidisers
5.2 Organic peroxides

Class 6

These materials are poisonous or infective.

Division 6.1 Poisons
6.2 Infective agents

Class 7

These are radioactive materials.

Class 8

These materials are corrosive.

Class 9

Miscellaneous hazardous substances.

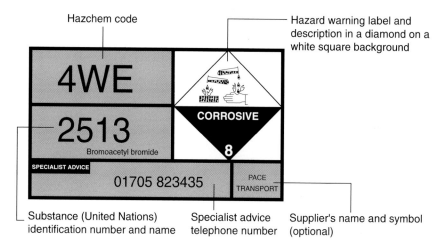

Figure 7.2 A UKTHIS sign.

The warning labels must give the following information:

- Hazchem scale number (or code)
- name of the substance and its United Nations (UN) code number
- UN hazard warning label
- specialist advice telephone number
- symbol or housemark of the manufacturer.

Hazchem scale

This gives the information necessary for the fire service to deal with the chemical (see Box 7.2).

The Hazchem code uses the letter 'E' to indicate that people should be warned to stay indoors with all doors and windows closed, but evacuation may need to be considered. Consult control centre, police and product expert. The letter 'V' means a product can be violently or even explosively reactive.

Hazchem scale card

This is a small card designed for fire service use that details the management of chemical spillages. A Hazchem scale card is carried in all fire appliances and should also be carried by all immediate care doctors and ambulances. They are available from The Stationery Office (Home Office 1999: Hazchem scale card, ISBN 0 11 341167 7).

Box 7.2 Hazchem scales

Recommended dispersal method

- jets
- fog
- foam
- dry agent.

Personal protection required:

- full body protective clothing with breathing apparatus
- breathing apparatus plus protective gloves.

Additional information

- the risk of explosion
- the need for evacuation
- the method of disposal:
  - may be diluted and washed down drains
  - should be prevented from entering drains or water course.

UN warning label

This is a diamond-shaped warning label (Fig. 7.3) indicating the primary hazard:

- inflammable
- corrosive
- toxic
- explosive.

If there is more than one hazard, the diamond will show an exclamation mark.

UN number

This number, which is used worldwide, is specific to individual substances so as to allow rapid identification.

Specialist advice telephone number

The 24-hour emergency telephone number of the supplier or manufacturer of the chemical is given on the label.

TREMCARD

This is a system developed by the European Council of Chemical Manufacturers Federation and is a manual of cards designed to give the emergency services information about dealing with chemicals, before expert advice can be obtained. The driver is supposed to keep the relevant TREMCARD in a locked pocket at the rear of the driver's seat. If the vehicle has a multiload, however, it can be difficult to know which of several TREMCARDs apply, and indeed what the consequences of mixing are. Drivers are also known to neglect or forget to change to the card appropriate for the current load. The TREMCARD is A4 sized and gives the following information:

- the correct British Standard chemical name of the substance;
- a description of the chemical's appearance and physical properties;
- the appropriate protection to be used;
- advice on the immediate management of spillage or fire;
- the first aid management of contaminated casualties.

ADR European transport system

This is a label borne on vehicles carrying hazardous substances to and from the European mainland. It is divided into two parts:

- the upper part displays the Kemler code;
- the lower part shows the UN number (Fig. 7.4).

The Kemler code   This is a numerical code using two or three digits that indicates the properties of the chemical. The first digit indicates the primary hazard and the next two digits any secondary hazard (see Box 7.3). An 'X' in front of the first number indicates that the product does not mix with water.

Box 7.3   The Kemler code

First digit:
 2 Gas
 3 Inflammable liquid
 4 Inflammable solid
 5 Oxidising substance or organic peroxide
 6 Toxic substance
 7 Radioactive substance
 8 Corrosive.

Second digit:
 0 No meaning
 1 Explosion risk
 2 Gas may be given off
 3 Inflammable risk
 5 Oxidising risk
 6 Toxic risk
 8 Corrosive risk
 9 Violent reaction risk

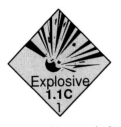

Class 1.1 - Mass explosion hazard

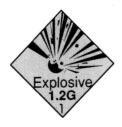

Class 1.2 - Projection hazard not mass explosion hazard

Class 1.4 Moderate explosion hazard

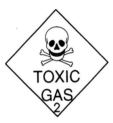

Class 2 - Toxic gas

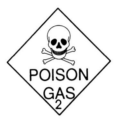

Class 3 - Flammable liquid

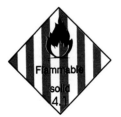

Class 4.1 - Flammable solid

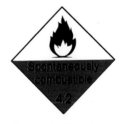

Class 4.2 - Spontaneously combustible substance

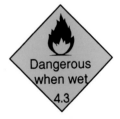

Class 4.3 - Dangerous when wet

Figure 7.3 Examples of UN warning labels.

Class 1.6 Minor
explosion hazard

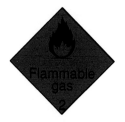

Class 2 - Flammable gas

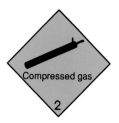

Class 2 - Non flammable
compressed gas

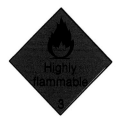

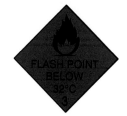

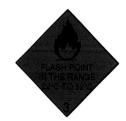

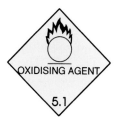

Class 5.1 - Oxidising
substance

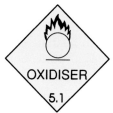

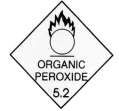

Class 5.2 - Organic peroxide

Figure 7.3 *Continued*

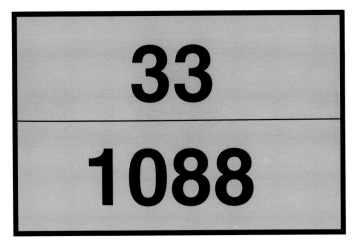

Figure 7.4 An ADR sign.

ACTION AT A CHEMICAL INCIDENT

The overriding principle must be that of the 1–2–3 of safety. That is:

personal safety – scene safety – casualty safety

in that order!

Doctors and paramedics are not immune to chemicals or radiation, and must stay away from contamination until the casualties are deemed safe by the fire service.

The UK Ambulance Service Association has recently developed guidelines on the management of causalities at chemical incidents (Department of Health 1998). The principle is that contaminated casualties will not be evacuated from the scene but will be decontaminated on site. This prevents vehicles as well as accident departments and their staff becoming contaminated. This raises the issue of how to decontaminate casualties as well as how to resuscitate them during that process. Increasingly counties have ambulance crew or immediate care doctors who are equipped or trained in the use of chemical protection clothing (Fig. 7.5). The fire service must however be responsible for all care to casualties before decontamination.

The new guidelines have many implications for training and new equipment. The question of chemical incidents first came onto the agenda around 1993. Regional health authorities set up working parties to determine areas of responsibilities between all the agencies involved in the many and varied aspects of a chemical incident. The outcome of these deliberations was published as Regional Guidelines.

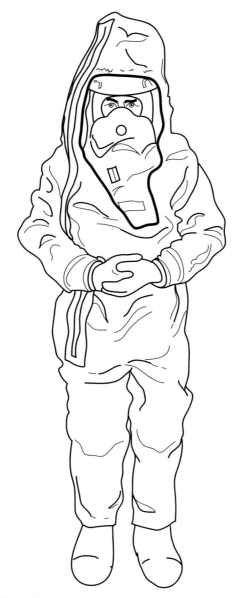

Figure 7.5   A fire service chemical protection suit.

In some counties, it was decided to take the Regional Guidelines further by producing more detailed documents. It is these that have been in operation over the past few years. Experience has shown that they do not satisfactorily deal with details; the subject of chemical incidents is therefore now high on the National Health Service (NHS) agenda.

The guidelines issued by the Ambulance Service Association to ambulance services are definitive (Department of Health 1998). These guidelines cover the areas of risk assessment, decontamination and personal protective equipment. This most sensible approach now needs to be taken forward into the field of the operational management of these incidents, both at the scene of the incident and at hospital accident and emergency (A&E) departments.

Chemical incident management

The usual perception of a chemical incident has become synonymous with fire, explosion and the emission of a cloud of toxic material resulting in many causalities. In reality, this is the 'worst case scenario'. Many incidents involve a single casualty or, at most, a handful.

For the same reasons the management of chemical incidents has been thought of as the prerogative of the fire service. Their expertise and experience in dealing with chemical incidents is second to none. They have access to Chem Data for information on firefighting and the protection of their staff (this is a computer database supplied to the fire service by the National Chemical Emergency Centre). This information, together with details of weather conditions from Chem-met, a collaboration between the Meteorological Office and the National Chemical Emergency Centre, enables some protection of the public in so far as the need to shelter or evacuate is concerned. These factors allow the fire service to discharge their responsibility, but the symptomatology, toxicology and urgent medical information in relation to minimum and maximum exposure levels is non-existent at the scene of an incident and is often only considered after the event.

While there are excellent systems for the longer-term management of these incidents from a medical point of view, response times to larger incidents from health professionals is understandably slow when compared with that of the emergency services. This type of medical response does not cater for the first hour of a live incident. For this reason, and because many chemical incidents do not involve the fire service, the ambulance service needs to make up these shortfalls.

By contacting the National Poisons Unit at a very early stage, every incident can be properly managed in a medical perspective from the outset. Procedures need to be in place to ensure that the resulting data are made readily available to A&E departments and nominated officers of the local health authority, irrespective of the size of the incident. Such a system is essential, bearing in mind the current legislation.

The Control of Substances Hazardous to Health (COSHH) Regulations 1989 (Department of the Environment, Transport and the Regions 1989) and the guidance from the Department of Health on the need to decontaminate and treat casualties who have been contaminated with chemicals places a duty of care on the ambulance service to ensure that safe systems of work are applied to persons involved in an incident and others who may be affected by it. This duty of care may extend to personnel from the other emergency services, A&E staff and the general public. It could also be argued that such an initial management system, with appropriate medical input, could ensure that only those requiring hospital treatment were actually taken to hospital, thus relieving a potentially enormous burden on A&E departments.

From an ambulance management point of view, it is essential that the response to a chemical incident is graded based on the information in the initial call, which is likely to come from a member of the public or the other emergency services. Dependent on the perceived severity of the incident, one or two levels of response would be initiated.

For a minor incident, domestic or industrial, a single ambulance would be dispatched to investigate. If the substance involved was known an immediate call would be made to the National Poisons Unit. The resulting information could be passed to the ambulance crews while en route to the scene in some instances, and would almost certainly be available by the time the crew reached the scene. All the available information would be passed to the local A&E department at an early stage. The crew would deal with the incident using set protocols, including updating ambulance control with relevant information from the scene, detailing the actual number of casualties and the substance involved. The duty control manager would evaluate this information and could send a supervisory officer and/or BASICS doctor to the scene if this was thought desirable. The National Poisons Unit would again be contacted if the information gained at the scene was different from that contained in the initial call and the new information passed on to the local A&E department.

The casualty(s) would be transported to the A&E department in a clean state when appropriate treatment and decontamination had been carried out at the scene. Incidents can occur where, although there is only a single casualty, there can be a danger of further casualties resulting from the decanting of the contents of one vehicle to another for the clean-up operation.

The ambulance service should maintain a presence at the scene until these operations were completed. The A&E department would be kept informed of progress and advised when the incident was closed. Where appropriate, advice would be sought from the National Poisons Unit and/or the occupational health department as to the need for any follow-up treatment for the crews involved.

Information gained for the crew would be made available to the other emergency service personnel. The ambulance service should also advise the appropriate director of public health immediately. The existing county procedures could be invoked by the A&E consultant, should he or she consider it appropriate.

Where the scenario was of a greater magnitude and where implications for the general public existed or were thought to exist, a much larger ambulance service response would be mounted from the outset. This would include the immediate mobilisation of supervisory officers, BASICS doctors and more sophisticated and larger decontamination facilities. A number of A&E departments would be alerted and the appropriate director of public health would be immediately informed by telephone. Information would be sought from the National Poisons Unit as previously described.

Decontamination: a realistic approach

In providing an A&E service, the ambulance service needs to deal with contamination on a regular basis. Contaminants come in many forms from deep mud found on building sites and at many sporting events to the heavy chemical or radiological contaminants found at registered chemical and nuclear sites. The spectrum is wide. Some contaminants are non-toxic and present no threat to the lives of casualty or rescuer, but may hinder effective treatment. Others are harmful and require very strict regimes to ensure the safety of ambulance staff and the best outcome possible for the casualty.

There may be wide variations in the number of casualties ranging from the single casualty to the mass casualty situation associated with larger releases of toxic material. The need for effective decontamination is, therefore, essential rather than a luxury.

The decontamination systems currently in place within many ambulance services, and in A&E departments, do not meet the requirements of existing legislation. The facilities available from the fire service are, almost invariably, high-pressure cold water jetting systems intended to wash down the outside of a chemical suit, not naked people. These facilities are of little use in the decontamination of seriously injured casualties and it could be argued that this process of decontamination could in some cases be more harmful to them than the contaminant. It is time for a totally new approach.

A protocol for decontamination has been documented recently by the working party set up by the Ambulance Service Association. The group has set standards for scene layout, personal protective clothing and decontamination procedures including water temperatures and the disposal of effluent where appropriate. It recommends that ambulance services carry out a risk assessment to determine the best arrangements for their particular area.

Such a risk assessment was undertaken by Lancashire. The conclusions were that no one form of decontamination regime would meet the needs of every incident. Requirements will vary depending upon the nature and toxicity of the contaminant, the number and severity of casualties, and the need to contain the resulting effluent and ensure a timely response to the incident. Standardising equipment, wherever possible, between the ambulance service and A&E departments is essential so that there can be inter-changeability of staff and equipment, joint training and, in consequence, less likelihood of accidents to all our staff. All these requirements need to be met in a cost-effective way given that the worst case scenario probably only occurs once in 30 years in the county.

First aid decontamination

Perhaps the most common requirement for decontamination arises from the single or dual casualty with non-toxic irritant contaminants. Such contaminants might include mud, petrol, spirit or the like. These are frequent occurrences for the ambulance service where decontamination, while not immediately essential in most cases, is desirable. This is because it prevents unnecessary irritation or discomfort to the casualty, and also the removal of mud, etc., enables a proper examination to take place. A small, self-contained battery-operated unit is available to fulfil this role. The unit consists of a hand-held shower unit, pump and water container. The unit could adequately provide full body decontamination for two casualties. There is no effluent containment and the unit uses cold water.

The provision of this unit on the immediate response vehicles provides a readily available response capable of meeting most needs. The water container can be filled with hot water at the start of each shift, thus providing hot water decontamination in line with the Ambulance Service Association recommendations. As the unit is portable it is capable of providing on-the-spot decontamination even in places that would otherwise be difficult to reach. The value of this unit is enhanced by full protective clothing being carried on the same vehicle, enabling toxic substances to be handled.

The capability of the unit is normally limited by the amount of water and the battery life. However, the unit can be plugged into the incubator supply point and the water can be topped up from hot water bottles, thus increasing the capability of the unit. The training requirement is negligible.

The unit would provide other unrelated facilities not currently catered for including eye irrigation and the provision of washing facilities for ambulance staff. All casualties would be presented at the A&E department in a much cleaner state than is currently possible. Even as a first response to a larger chemical incident, the unit could be selectively used to decont-aminate casualties most at risk until more appropriate arrangements could be put in place.

Decontamination for larger incidents

The Ambulance Service Association recommendations for mass decontam-ination are many and varied but basically require a shelter through which ambulant or stretcher cases can receive appropriate supervised hot water decontamination based on the dirty-to-clean side traverse of the casualty (Fig. 7.6). The effluent needs to be contained and, preferably, pumped away from the shelter to minimise the build up of fumes. An inflatable shelter has been produced that is adequate for the perceived risk in many counties. The shelter is inflated by compressed gas and requires no maintenance of pressure once inflated. Leaks are not immediately catastrophic, as there is time to take remedial action before total collapse of the shelter. The base of the structure forms a catch well that has pipes at each corner through which the effluent can be pumped away. The provision makes the unit suit-

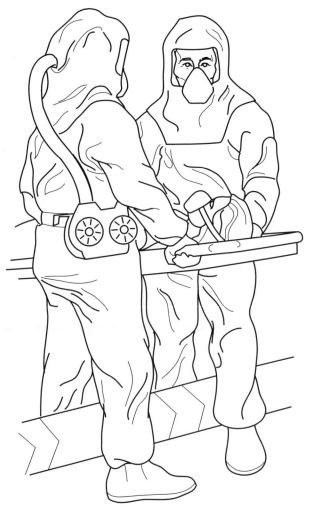

Figure 7.6 Chemical protection clothing suitable for ambulance and medical personnel involved in decontamination of casualties.

able for use on uneven terrain, as only one pipe is required to remove the volume of effluent generated. The unit can be inflated in about 2 minutes on either hard or soft standing as required, and by one person if necessary.

To be assured of a realistic response time of 30 minutes throughout the county, most ambulance services would require approximately three units. For counties with a more significant risk of a chemical incident there is a larger Swedish unit currently available. There is however a need to provide a tow vehicle and trained drivers, and the unit in general is less manageable. Furthermore, one of the problems identified in rigid units with fixed piping is the risk of residual water from poor drainage technique freezing during storage in cold weather and rendering the unit inoperative for some time.

For a mobile unit there are three problems that are not resolved: the provision of hot water, lighting and water supply. The latter two are not a problem as lighting can be provided from the parent vehicle or by use of a small generator. The water supply can come from a hydrant or fire tender. The more problematic area is that of providing hot water. It is possible to use through-flow water heaters fueled by bottled gas. The unit needs to be permanently mounted in an equipment vehicle to which a water supply would be piped. A single outlet would then carry hot water to a maximum of four showerheads located within each shelter.

At larger incidents several units could be deployed simultaneously, providing maximum throughput of casualties, and the units could be configured to provide separate facilities for ambulant and stretcher cases or to separate males from females. The flexibility would exist to provide decontamination facilities at two separate locations if the geography of an incident dictated. Alternatively, the unit could be deployed to a site remote from the actual incident such as a rest centre.

It also enables the provision of a facility for casualties who might self-refer to a minor injuries unit, not having decontamination facilities or the trained staff, rather than to a listed A&E department. Indeed, directing casualties to such a unit may be desirable in order to relieve pressure on A&E, provided that decontamination could be provided.

Unfortunately, at the current time, different counties are pursuing different options. Standardisation in techniques and equipment used in decontamination has many advantages. The training costs would be minimised because everyone could operate to the same protocols in terms of unit operation, the decontamination of casualties, the bagging and labelling of property and the decontamination of the equipment after use. It would also make it possible to interchange staff, both at the scene and at hospitals. Where common systems exist each can learn from the other and reduce accidents. The ability to train together would be enhanced and more meaningful. At a practical level it is possible for hospitals to assist one another. Should the single unit available prove inadequate, units could be loaned from hospitals or ambulance services not involved in the incident.

RADIATION HAZARDS

Memories of the Cold War and Chernoble, mingled with science fiction, have created an exceptional misunderstanding of radiation in many members of the general public. In reality, radiation is no different from any other toxic substance. Understanding the nature of the substance is the key to its safe handling.

Radiation is the process by which energy is transferred from its source to other objects. Heat is radiated from a fire, light is radiated from a torch, and radio waves are radiated from a mobile phone. This section concentrates on the 'ionising radiation' from radioactive sources. A radiation hazard is labelled with the symbol shown in Figure 7.7.

Radiation is not new. The earth is exposed continuously to the radiation from the sun and the stars (cosmic radiation), but most of it is absorbed by the ozone layer and atmosphere. Flying in aircraft increases your exposure to this radiation, but staying on the ground has its hazards too. Marie Curie extracted radium from naturally occurring pitchblende. Natural deposits of radioactive minerals in rock produce radon gas that accumulates in houses, acting as a significant source of radiation exposure to the local population (in the UK areas of higher radon exposure are Cornwall and Aberdeen). We are also exposed to radiation whenever we have a dental or

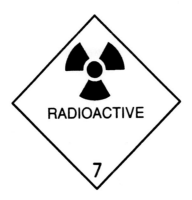

Class 7 - Radioactive substance

Figure 7.7 Radiation hazard symbol.

medical X-ray. It is the degree of exposure to radiation that determines the effect it will have on someone's health.

Radioactive materials may be solids, liquids or gases. Although they look no different from any other solid, liquid or gas, they do emit two types of particle and two types of radiation.

Alpha particles

These are the largest of the particles emitted by a radioactive source, and also the least dangerous external radiation. They travel only a few millimetres and are stopped by paper, clothing and skin. They can only enter the body by inhalation, injection or ingestion. Once within the body, however, they will interfere with chemical processes and damage internal organs. Internal exposure to alpha particles is considered the most serious form of radiation exposure.

Beta particles

These are 7000 times smaller than alpha particles but have more energy and therefore considerably more penetrating power. They can be stopped by thick clothing or thin layers of metal or masonry. When concentrated they can cause burns to unprotected skin, and, like alpha particles, are obviously dangerous if they become internal to the body through inhalation or ingestion.

Gamma rays

Gamma rays have 10 000 times the penetration power of alpha particles and 100 times the power of beta particles. Protective clothing does not stop gamma rays. They can produce both localised burns and extensive internal damage.

X-rays

X-rays and gamma rays are similar in that they are very penetrating and can pass through the body. They cannot be stopped but can be absorbed by shielding, can be reduced by increasing the distance from the source, and reduce by time as the half-life of the source is reached.

Protection against radiation

With both types of radiation, the key to protection lies in:

D density of material between you and the source;
D distance from the source (inverse square law, Fig. 7.8);
T time duration of exposure.

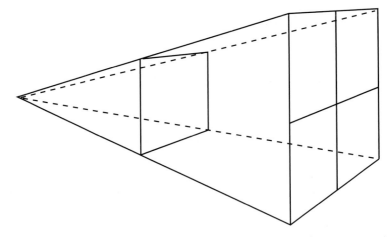

Figure 7.8 Radiation reduces with distance; double the distance reduces exposure to a quarter.

The danger from ingested materials is that some of the radioactive isotopes involved tend to concentrate in certain organs of the body where elements with similar properties are found. For example, radioactive iodine-131 tends to concentrate in the thyroid gland. In 1986 Polish children were given potassium iodate tablets with the intention of saturating the gland so that any radioactive iodine would be rejected by the body and excreted. This is also part of the policy for handling radioactive leaks in the UK. Following a radioactive leak at Sellafield many years ago, thousands of gallons of milk had to be discarded as cows eating the grass would absorb strontium–90, which could enter the food chain and be utilised in the same way as calcium, being laid down in bone.

Effects on the human body

Exposure to gamma or X-radiation does not make an object radioactive. It is only the presence of a radioactive source as a residue that poses a threat to rescuers.

Huge amounts of radiation will cause death very quickly. The cellular damage in the nervous system causes cerebral oedema, with loss of consciousness and coma.

Lesser amounts of radiation will cause damage to any cells that divide rapidly, for example cells in the bone marrow and intestine. The most immediate effects are related to these organs. Nausea, vomiting and diarrhoea, bleeding and loss of resistance to infection are the results of large exposure. Provided these effects can be effectively managed, and no further exposure occurs, the person will recover. There can be long-term effects, however, because the risk of cancer in irradiated tissue is increased substantially.

Measurement of radiation

The amount of emitted radiation is expressed in a variety of different values. Radiation intensity is measured in becquerels (Bq), and the absorbed dose is measured in centigrays per hour. A quality factor needs to be applied to arrive at a dose equivalent. The figures are 1 for X-rays, gamma rays and beta particles, 10 for neutrons and 20 for alpha particles. The dose equivalent is measured in millisieverts. An annual exposure of 2 millisieverts occurs from natural radiation, or from a single chest X-ray.

Radiation exposure is determined by the reading on a personal dosimeter. A dosimeter can be a piece of photographic film, which is exposed by radiation and fogs, or it may be an electrostatic device. Dosimeters have to be worn before exposure occurs, during the entire exposure, and read after reaching a secure environment.

A body can compensate for an exposure of 200 centigrays over a few minutes but the repair process required to compensate for the damage caused by this exposure cannot resist a dose in excess of 15 centigrays a day. A 600 centigray dose will kill 50% of those exposed to it.

KEY POINTS

- Exposure to radiation does not make a casualty radioactive.
- Casualties contaminated by radioactive particles need decontamination.
- Radioactive particles are dangerous if inhaled or ingested.
- Exposure to radiation is limited by density, distance and time (DDT).

BIOLOGICAL HAZARDS

Biological hazards are numerous. The casualty can potentially be a biohazard by having hepatitis, syphilis or human immune deficiency virus. These are routine hazards every health care worker should be familiar with and will not be discussed further. Emergency personnel should also be disciplined in the safe disposal of needles and scalpel blades so that needlestick injuries are minimised. Always be aware of the danger that medical sharps can be overlooked, however. An intravenous cannula is available that automatically sheaths the needle, and these are particularly suitable for the prehospital environment. Broken glass and metal also are capable of causing an injury that allows inoculation to take place.

Biological hazards such as bacterial cultures or clinical waste are transported to and from laboratories, surgeries and incinerators on a daily basis. They should be clearly marked with the biohazard symbol (Fig. 7.9).

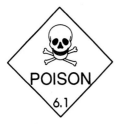

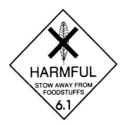

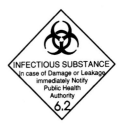

Class 6.1 Group A - Toxic   Class 6.1 Group B - Harmful   Class 6.2 - Infectious
substance   substance   substance

Figure 7.9   Biological hazard symbols.

Accidents involving the spillage of clinical waste must be governed by a knowledge of the likely organisms. The management of a spilt anthrax culture is obviously different from that of a puddle of patient's urine. Dangerous micro-organisms are not always found with international warning symbols attached, however. The dangers of sewerage are obvious, and emergency crews would probably be cautious about funeral parlours, certain areas in abattoirs and similar clearly high-risk areas. However, the risk of Weil's disease from areas where rats may urinate, and the water courses that drain them, may not be common knowledge. Every year canoeists and windsurfers contract the disease. There is even an uncertain risk from opening graves from the Georgian era, which may contain small-pox or plague victims.

Certain environments can carry airborne organisms. These include farmer's lung from mouldy hay, psittacosis from diseased birds such as pigeons, and most seriously anthrax from imported animal hides.

Scabies, fleas and lice are almost occupational hazards for emergency service personnel dealing with vagrants. But it is also possible to contract ringworm and orf from having to handle animals to reach the casualty. Certain areas of forestry, in particular the New Forest, have deer tics that carry Lyme disease. Sheep tics are equally unpleasant guests to acquire from a farm rescue.

Risks can arise with domestic animals, farm animals and wild animals. The most common danger from pets is the dog that is trying to protect its sick owner. These animals respond well to your concern for their master. A more dangerous situation is the dog that sees the casualty as its prize of war and will fight to keep it from you. If time allows the RSPCA (Royal Society for the Prevention of Cruelty to Animals) should be contacted to restrain the animal, or a local vet to sedate or destroy it. The response from these individuals may not be as rapid as necessary and the possibility of using the armed police response unit should be considered. If there is an immediate risk to life then firefighters, with the insulation in their garments providing protection, and armed with hoses or devices such as a Hooligan tool, can usually drive the animal away from the casualty. In the USA and Canada it is possible to purchase pepper spray to repel dogs and bears and the police pepper spray will serve as effectively. There is anecdotal evidence that CS spray has a reduced effect on dogs and probably should not be tried. Exotic pets can create problems as well. Most pet snakes are non-venomous, but tarantulas have recently been discovered to be able to fire their barbed leg hairs into the eyes of people who hold them. Three people have been reported as having severely reduced vision from the reaction that results.

Farm animals can frequently behave in unpredictable manners when frightened. Overturned vehicles carrying animals can pose serious threats if the animals are released. Escaping animals can run wild on the road, causing other road users to act irrationally. Larger animals can cause serious injury if they stampede. If they are trapped they can bite and kick rescuers.

Animals don't have to be involved in road accidents to become frightened. The horse that throws its rider and the bull that gores a farmer are all likely to behave unpredictably and need a trained handler. Wild animals can often be the cause of motorway accidents, particularly deer. If the opportunity affords itself (because the beast is stunned) it should be tethered safely on as short a tether as possible. Do not fasten it to a vehicle because if it does become aggressive, considerable damage can be done.

Safari parks and zoos pose special risks, but at least there are handlers rapidly available who are skilled in handling the animals. It is essential that the handlers control the animal before an approach to the casualty is made.

Plants are not totally benign either. The Giant Hogweed is probably the most dangerous of the plants that grow in the UK (Fig. 7.10). Growing 10–12 feet (3–4 m) tall along river banks and in damp areas, this hollow-stemmed plant has fine bristles and a sap that causes blistering and prolonged photosensitivity. It has caused blindness in dogs. Children find great pleasure in cutting down these large plants and will use them to construct dens as they are lightweight. If faced with entering a hogweed patch, all exposed skin should be covered, and as soon as possible the clothing changed and skin washed.

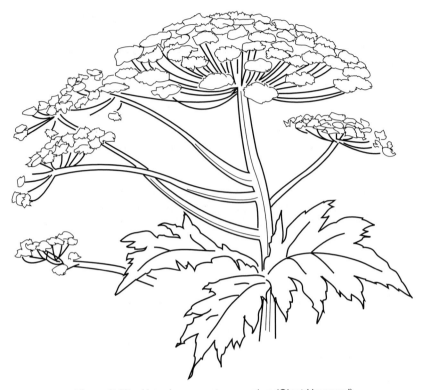

Figure 7.10 *Heracleum mantegazzanium* (Giant Hogweed).

Self-test questions for Chapter 7

1. What information does a United Kingdom Transport Hazard Information System (UKTHIS) plate carry?

2. Where would you expect to find the UKTHIS plate on a vehicle?

3. What Hazchem symbol means evacuation should be considered?

4. What is the 1–2–3 of safety?

5. Who is responsible for casualties that are contaminated?

6. What are the major categories of hazardous substances?

7. A casualty is covered with an unknown dry chemical powder in a laboratory accident. Is it safe to transport him to hospital provided the ambulance crew only touch him while wearing gloves? If not, why not?

8. A lorry does not carry a UKTHIS plate but does have a plate with an upper number and a lower number. What are these numbers and what do they mean?

9. What are the ambulance service responsibilities at a chemical incident?

10. What are the various forms of ionising radiation?

11. State the factors that affect the radiation dose an individual might receive.

12. List 10 biological hazards that can be present at an accident scene.

13. What are the key elements of a good first report to control?

Answers on p. 207.

8

Fire safety

Fire is an oxidation reaction that releases chemical energy in the form of heat and light. Flames actually occur in the vapour that is released from the fuel. Depending on the type of fuel, this vapour is already present or is released when the material is heated. Fire, therefore, can only exist in the presence of three factors:

- fuel
- heat
- oxygen.

Fire is fought by depriving the fire of one of these three factors. This can be achieved by removing the fuel, such as turning off the gas to a gas fire or creating a fire break in a forest fire. Alternatively, the heat may be removed by using water, which requires huge amounts of energy before it is converted to steam. Finally, the fire may be deprived of oxygen, for example by putting a damp cloth over a burning chip pan.

Different fuels require different methods of management, and there are different types of extinguisher. To identify the appropriate extinguisher for the fuel they are classified into four types. These fuel types are described below.

CLASSES OF FUEL

Class A: Carbonaceous

This type includes coal, coke, wood, cotton, paper, straw, etc., and is the most common fuel type in the environment. Significant heat needs to be applied to these materials to create a vapour phase. For this reason the most effective method of extinguishing this type of fire is by cooling with water.

Class B: Liquids and solids that become liquids

Liquids have to have a vapour phase to ignite: if they are too cold to create a vapour above them, then they will not ignite. When the temperature is raised to the flashpoint the vapour will ignite in the presence of a flame, but will be extinguished if the external flame is removed. At the fire point a brief exposure to a flame will create a fire that continues after the flame has been removed. Brandy has to be warmed to achieve an adequate vapour before it will ignite, as every Christmas pudding chef can testify. Brake fluid has a fire point lower than the temperature of a hot exhaust manifold. At a temperature known as the spontaneous combustion point the thermal energy in the vapour is so great that it spontanously bursts into flame. The concentration of the gas with oxygen is critical: if it is too low, then there is not enough gas to act as fuel; and if it is too much, then there is insufficient oxygen to support combustion.

Class C: Gases

Apart from domestic gas, many homes will have portable gas heaters with gas cylinders. On a smaller scale, inflammable gases are increasingly found in domestic aerosols that purport to be 'ozone friendly – CFC free'. This results in gases such as butane being commonly found in canisters in the home. Domestic aerosol cans will explode if overheated – and this does not necessarily require a fire. There are many cases where the can was left on an electric storage heater, which, when it charges overnight, heats the can to the critical temperature. The can is designed with several pressure-release devices. They do not always work before the can explodes. Frequently, however, two 'plink' sounds will be heard as the expansion joints operate. At an uncertain time afterwards the end blows off and the flammable gas has the opportunity of igniting. Large butane storage cylinders for building heating systems are actually sited with a safe trajectory considered into the location.

Acetylene cylinders pose particular problems when they become over-heated as they can develop hot spots that can cause explosions many hours after the original fire has been put out.

If a gas leak has ignited it is best to contain the effect of the flame, but it should not be extinguished unless the source can be turned off. To extinguish the flame would otherwise allow an explosive quantity to accumulate, thus increasing the danger.

If you smell domestic gas then you should not operate any electrical switches or equipment that is not 'intrinsically safe'. To do so could cause an explosion. Obviously do not allow people to smoke. If possible seek the stop valve beside the gas meter and turn it from being in line with the pipe to right angles to it. Ventilate the area, leave the premises and call out the Transco Gas Engineers on 0800 111999. Gas can accumulate in loft spaces and other building cavities and may not disperse very quickly. As you ventilate the premises they may cool and there is the risk that a thermostat will operate electrical equipment automatically. The danger is not over until the experts have deemed the property safe.

Class D: Metals

Metals may not seem to be the type of material that will burn, but lathe turnings, or swarf as it is known, can burn. Magnesium and aluminium both burn quite easily. There is very little flame and it may be supposed that the fire can be extinguished easily. This is true but it must be done with dry sand as the heat of fire is so great that water is broken down into its constituent parts of hydrogen and oxygen, thus increasing the intensity of the combustion. Magnesium is found as an alloy in sports car wheels, and also in the cylinder blocks of some cars.

Previously there was another class of fire listed, that being electrical fires. This has now been removed as electricity is of course a source of ignition but is not a fuel source for fire itself. Once the electricity is turned off the fire will only continue if it has a fuel type to burn. The danger of electrical fires is that the electric current will run to earth through the liquid jet to the extinguisher and electrocute the operator. Water and dry powder also do untold damage to electrical components and therefore carbon dioxide extinguishers are preferred not only for their safety, but also for their damage limitation capability.

Fire extinguishers are designed to fight fires of a particular type. On the extinguisher the rating for each type of fuel will be found. Generally any medium that can extinguish class D fires can also extinguish class A, B and C fires, but a medium that can extinguish class A fires may be unsuitable on B, C and D.

BASIC FIRE SAFETY

Remember that fire is best prevented. When called to incidents bear in mind that the emergency that resulted in your call may have distracted someone from watching over a fire hazard or may have created a fire hazard that needs to be made safe. The choking child may have distracted a parent from the chip pan. The wife may have put clothes in front of the fire as she ran to help her husband when he fell. The plumber may have left his blow torch on when his mate fell through the ceiling. The leaking petrol line may be near a sparking wire. You may be about to turn on the light to find the source of the gas leak.

If you suspect fire don't walk in unaware. Merely opening the door can give fire the oxygen it needs – read the section on backdraught and flashover later in this chapter. Always feel the temperature of doors before you open them. Look at the windows as you arrive; with potential backdraught scenarios you can get the explosively inflammable gases condensing on the glass as a black oily film. If attending a fire in a block of flats avoid the lift, but even if you do use it **always** go to the floor below and ascend the last flight of stairs carefully – you don't want to put yourself into a cremator once the doors open.

If you must enter a smoke-filled area keep low – smoke is hot air and rises. Be wary of stairs and floors above a fire; they may be seriously weakened, so keep to the edges where possible. If you must penetrate a fire to effect a rescue, realise that it is easier to get in than it is to get out, particularly if you find the casualty. The fire will have got worse, you will have got tired and affected by fumes, and there is the added load of the casualty. Think very, very hard before you try to do the work of the trained firefighter wearing breathing apparatus, who, in the UK, will be very quickly behind you.

PRACTICAL USE OF PORTABLE FIRE EXTINGUISHERS

There are some basic rules that must apply to the use of fire extinguishers. They are principles that are so basic to firefighting that you should never consider using an extinguisher without following each and every one of them (Box 8.1). Your life could depend upon it.

Fire extinguishers may contain any one of a variety of firefighting media. Recent European legislation requires all extinguishers to be red, but up to 5% of the extinguisher may be in a colour that identifies the contents. The appropriate colours are red for water, cream for foam, blue for dry powder,

---

Box 8.1   Rules for using fire extinguishers

Rule 1   Always summon help first.

Rule 2   Choose an appropriate fire extinguisher.

Rule 3   Test the extinguisher before you return to the fire.

Rule 4   Never allow the fire between you and your exit.

Rule 5   Use the extinguisher as far from the fire as possible.

Rule 6   Never turn your back on a fire.

Rule 7   Know when to get out because the fire is winning.

black for carbon dioxide, and more rarely found these days, green for BCF. Extinguishers are also powered either by a carbon dioxide cartridge or by direct pressurisation. Those directly pressurised will always have a pressure gauge, as in Figure 8.1, and those with a cartridge will usually have a wider neck to accommodate it. On this type the hose and trigger are attached by a plastic screw thread. This has been known to fail and therefore wide neck extinguishers should never be pressurised with the operator standing over it.

The most suitable for Class A fires is water, which is cheap and provides good cooling, thus reducing the risk of re-ignition. However, water is an electrical conductor, which makes it unsuitable for electrical fires. It will also make Class B fires considerably worse by giving the liquid a medium on which it can float and by creating an aerosol of steam and burning fuel. To achieve maximum cooling effect the jet should be directed into the heart of the fire. One of the problems firefighters can have with the first use of water is the blast of steam that blows back at them.

An alternative is foam, which puts Class B fires out by starving them of oxygen. Although foam acts slowly, once the fire is out it has the maximum

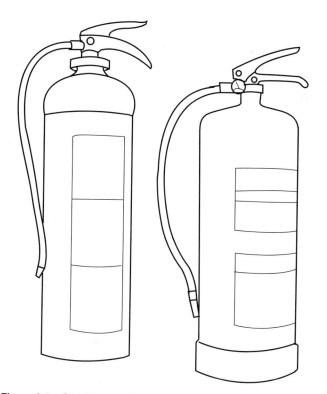

Figure 8.1 Cartridge type (left) and pressurised (right) extinguishers.

chance of keeping it out. Foam is of several varieties. Aspirated foam has a special design of nozzle (or branch) through which air is entrained by the Venturi effect into an animal protein solution. Ideally the jet is directed onto a vertical surface behind the fire and the foam allowed to flow over the liquid (Fig. 8.2). Alternatively the foam is allowed to rain onto the fire, or can even be bounced off the ground in front of the fire. It is important to reduce the velocity at which the foam escapes by these techniques so as to prevent it from being thrust into the liquid and contaminated by it. Always empty the extinguisher to produce a foam blanket of maximum thickness. Never use dry powder after a foam extinguisher as the powder will cause the foam to disintegrate. A popular extinguisher uses aqueous film-forming foam (AFFF). While marked as a foam extinguisher it has no branch on the hose and the foam falls as a spray. The film created is easily disrupted and re-ignition can occur.

Some Class B fires may be caused by polar solvents such as methanol. Methanol is used as a fuel in some racing cars, particularly on speed trials, and is also used to clean pipes on gas rigs. It burns with an invisible flame unless contaminated by impurities. Dry powder is an excellent source of

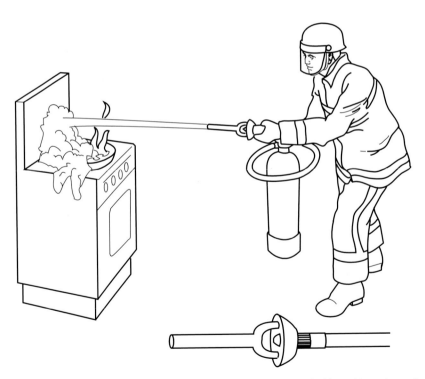

Figure 8.2 Aspirated foam extinguisher in use. The inset shows the Venturi branch used on aspirated foam extinguishers.

impurities. If ordinary foam is used on a methanol fire the foam rapidly deteriorates due to the absorption of the water content. Alcoseal is the appropriate foam for this sort of fire and should be available wherever these fuels are to be found.

Carbon dioxide is the best choice for electrical fires, not only because it doesn't conduct electricity but also because it doesn't cause further damage to the electrical apparatus (Fig. 8.3). It is very noisy in use and frost damage may occur if you touch the horn while it is in use. A carbon dioxide extinguisher should always be carried with the base in the left hand, and the trigger operated by the right hand. This keeps the horn away from the face. A concentration of 30% has to be achieved before the fire is extinguished so the fire compartment should be afforded minimum ventilation. Carbon dioxide at 30% is not respirable so exposure to concentrated gas should be minimised. The pitch of the noise it makes changes distinctly as

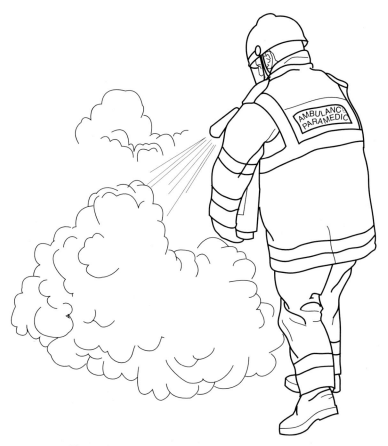

Figure 8.3 Using a carbon dioxide (CO_2) extinguisher.

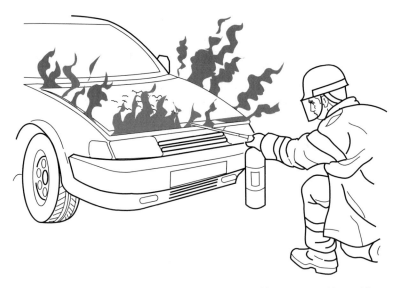

Figure 8.4 A BCF extinguisher sprayed into this released but unopened bonnet to extinguish a car engine fire.

the gas is about to run out. Carbon dioxide extinguishers do not last for long; the average extinguisher has less than a minute's worth of gas inside.

Dry powder is often bicarbonate of soda. It has a rapid knockdown effect and is not toxic to the environment or to humans, but has little cooling power and thus fires can easily restart. The powder interferes with the chemical process of combustion and therefore needs to be directed into the vapour phase of the fuel. A rapid sweeping process is required to sweep the fire from the fuel. As the powder forces its way towards the fire the pressure wave of air ahead often causes a flare up of the fire. In a confined space be wary of the flame rolling over and behind you.

A choice that is becoming less common is BCF, which is excellent for fires but not for the environment (Fig. 8.4). BCF is also degraded in fire and becomes highly toxic to both people and animals. It is therefore no longer on sale, but is still found in many vehicles that were fitted with extinguishers when purchased.

USING A FIRE BLANKET

Fire blankets are usually 1 metre square, although 2 metre by 1 metre blankets are available and suitable for people on fire. Blankets are ideal for chip pan fires, and require only confidence and a little training to use successfully. The blanket should be held to protect the hands and the face. The blanket should be kept on the exit route from the kitchen, or with a fire extinguisher beside the telephone. The blanket is opened out in front of you. Take an edge between both thumbs and forefingers, with the hands about 18 inches (45 cm) apart, palms uppermost. Then, still gripping the blanket, turn the palms downwards. This should bring the sides of the blanket over the hands and forearms to protect them (Stage 1 in Fig. 8.5). Keeping your arms out in front of you, advance carefully towards the fat fire, avoiding any fat spilt on the floor, and carefully and deliberately lay the blanket over the pan (Stage 2 in Fig. 8.5). Tuck the edges in and turn off

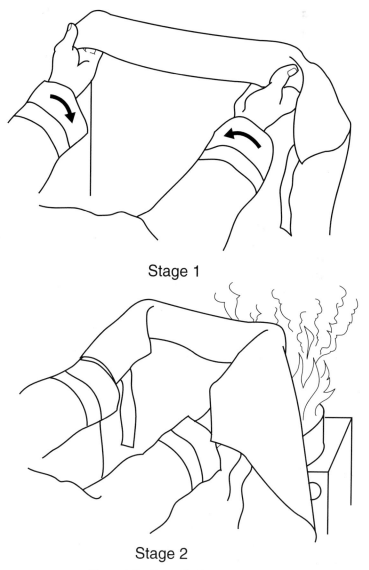

Stage 1

Stage 2

Figure 8.5   How to hold a fire blanket.

the fuel supply to the cooker. Call the fire service to deal with the hot fat. If the blanket is removed it will re-ignite. Do not try to move the chip pan as the fire will have weakened the handle joint and it may well fail as you carry the pan.

Deaths still regularly occur when people throw water on chip pan fires. The water sinks to the bottom of the hot oil and becomes steam at nearly 400°C, expanding to 1700 times its original volume. This explosive expansion produces a cloud of nebulised flaming oil that rolls through the kitchen, igniting any flammable material in its path.

BACKDRAUGHT AND FLASHOVER

Flashover has been long known to the fire service. It occurs when the temperature of a contained but ventilated space reaches the point where the fabric of the room spontaneously ignites.

Backdraught is a phenomenon that has become increasingly common since the introduction of modern building techniques. With double glazing, cavity wall insulation, draught excluders and a lack of chimneys because of central heating the modern house, owing to its lack of ventilation, is prone to both condensation and backdraught.

Backdraught occurs when a compartment of a building has a fire within it. The temperature of the room rises until flashover would occur were it not for the shortage of oxygen within the compartment. The superheated and potentially explosive gases, with oxygen to sustain the fire, start to cool, and in doing so suck more air into the compartment. This fuels the fire and the gases then expand again. This process is repeated, causing a pattern of smoke generation likened to breathing. At the door there may be a whistling noise as air is sucked in, and the door will be hot, particularly the handle. At the window the hot gases will start to condense, producing deposits.

Depending on the degree to which there is still flame within the room one of two consequences may result if the compartment is entered. If the fire is still vigorous the door may be sucked open by the in-rush of air. The ensuing upsurge in combustion then causes a rapid expansion of gas that may slam the door shut and the explosion will follow. The explosion may be the first thing that happens. If, however, the fire has died to a smoulder, more time will be needed before the gases ignite. The danger comes not on opening the door – indeed, in one case a person in the room had been removed by one firefighter while another two continued to fight the fire. When the backdraught occurred the door was slammed shut on the hose, jamming it shut, with the loss of the two lives.

The dangers are not merely confined to the room that contains the fire. The explosive gas mixture may escape from the room and mix with air. Now cooler and away from an ignition source, it will wait for a flame or spark to explode.

The danger of backdraught is its unpredictability, and modern practice is to ventilate the compartment in a controlled manner. The aim is to create ventilation high in the room and then low down. There is the danger of an explosion and instantaneous flashover but at least the fire can then be fought in a safe and conventional manner.

KEY POINTS

- Always summon help first.
- Choose an appropriate fire extinguisher.
- Test the extinguisher before you return to the fire.
- Never allow the fire between you and your exit.
- Use the extinguisher as far from the fire as possible.
- Never turn your back on a fire.
- Know when to get out because the fire is winning.

Self-test questions for Chapter 8

1. Give the seven rules governing the use of a fire extinguisher.
2. The nearest extinguisher to a frying pan fire has a black label on it. Can it be used and how will you know it's nearly empty?
3. What would happen if the label were red?
4. What is flashover?
5. What are the conditions that predispose to backdraught?
6. What are the four types of fuel?
7. What might warn you of a backdraught in the making?
8. Give two disadvantages of BCF as a firefighting medium.
9. Give three reasons why it is inadvisable to enter a smoke-filled area to rescue a casualty.
10. Name three types of foam extinguisher.
11. What sort of fire extinguisher can cause a flare-up when it is first operated?

Answers on p. 208.

Electrical safety

Since the dawn of time humans have been fascinated by lightning and static electricity. Even in modern society there is still portrayal of electricity as the bringer of life, or death, in films and fiction. Electricity is like any other aspect of natural science: it can be a threat to life if handled incautiously. Fatalities and injuries still occur too frequently, in spite of, or possibly because of, its almost universal presence at work and in the home.

To be able to work safely with electricity certain principles need to be understood. Atoms are commonly represented like little solar systems with a central nucleus like the sun, consisting of neutrons and positively charged protons, surrounded by orbiting negatively charged electrons. If an atom loses an electron it carries a net positive charge, and an atom with an electron surplus to requirements carries a net negative charge. Electrons will try to migrate to a positively charged atom, and will do so if the material between them will permit this. Some materials, such as metal and water, enable this transfer of electrons and are known as electrical conductors. Other materials prevent this transfer and are known as insulators. The ability to resist the flow of electrons depends upon the amount of force encouraging them to move. This is known as the electromotive force and is measured in volts. The electromotive force used in domestic mains electricity in the UK is 250 volts.

The number of electrons that actually flows along a conductor at any given moment is called the current, and is comparable to the current of water in a pipe. Current is measured in amperes. Thus an electrical appliance plug fuse is rated for the number of amperes of current it can carry before it melts and stops the current. The amount of work available from an electrical supply is measured in watts. The number of watts is calculated by multiplying the voltage by the amperage. Thus a 13 amp 250 volt plug can supply 3250 watts. This means it is suitable for a 3 kilowatt heater.

Electricity can be used to generate heat and light by applying enough voltage to a current to force it through a material that is either too long, too narrow, or too poor a conductor for its easy passage. These materials are deemed to have a high resistance to electricity. Resistance is measured in ohms. An example of resistance is found with loudspeakers. They are often marked as 8 or 16 Ω (ohms).

Electrical current with sufficient voltage to use animal tissue as a conductor has two effects. First, the tissues act like any other resistance and becomes heated. The burns from electrical current may appear to be confined to where the current made contact but in fact they can penetrate deeply in an ever-widening cone as the current seeks a broad path to earth. Second, because of the use of electric potentials by nerves and muscles, an electrical shock can disrupt muscle and nerve function. This can cause hand muscles to clamp a grip onto the source, paralyse muscle and nerve function, and cause cardiac arrhythmias including ventricular fibrillation.

STATIC ELECTRICITY

When two dissimilar objects that are relative insulators are rubbed together electrons can be ripped from one and attached to the other. When the voltage is in excess of around 400 volts a spark is created as electrons flow across the air gap between the surfaces. The perceived shock is slight as the actual current is very small.

Static electricity is commonly only a nuisance, but it can become dangerous in certain environments. Certain helicopters generate large amounts of static electricity as the rotor blades sweep through the air. The Sea King is a particular example. When a winch line is lowered it must be allowed to touch either land or water before being handled or the shock received as the current passes to earth will be significant. Aircraft can generate static electricity as they fly through the air. When refuelling aircraft, tankers will make connection to the aircraft with an earthing cable to prevent static electricity sparks causing a fuel vapour explosion. Operating theatre equipment is 'grounded' to prevent static electricity causing explosions in an oxygen and anaesthetic gas-rich atmosphere. Computer engineers will attach themselves to computer equipment with a 'grounding lead' to prevent static destroying delicate circuits. If you are advised that you are in a risk area, you should take advice with regard to clothing, avoid use of any electrical equipment that is not intrinsically safe (including radios, radiopagers and defibrillators), and obviously be wary about the use of oxygen.

LIGHTNING

The most impressive example of static electricity on earth has to be lightning. Around the world each day there are an average of 3000 thunderstorms with lightning striking the planet at around 100 times a second. There are an average of 300 000 lightning strikes on the British Isles each year, with June, July, August and September being the peak months. Huge static electricity charges are built up by the swirling actions of the air currents. Each discharge of electricity releases a current of around 200 000 amperes with a force of 50 000 000 volts. The temperature of lightning is around 30 000°C but lasts for only a few thousandths of a second. The probability of being hit by lightning is estimated at 1 in 3 million. This is fives times more likely than winning the lottery. Direct hits will kill, and every year nearly 2000 people die worldwide from lightning strikes. The death toll in the UK is low, averaging about five people per year. Of those who die about 30% die in open fields or recreation areas and parks, 17% die from sheltering under trees, 13% from being on or near water, 6% from being on or near tractors, 4% from being on golf courses and 1% from talking on mobile phones in the open.

About 70% of those struck by lightning survive, because fortunately the path to earth is not solely through the victim. The person who is struck is caught in only part of the lightning strike, and it often arcs over the body's surface rather than passing through it. This surface effect accounts for the bizarre fern leaf burns, destruction of clothing and the strange way in which the shoes are often blown off. This is due to the fact that the surface charge meets an increase in resistance at seams within the leather and between the uppers and the soles. This increase in resistance causes heat that burns through the stitching. The current that flows through the body flows along blood vessels and the cerebrospinal fluid. The brain stem centre controlling breathing is most affected because the cerebrospinal fluid pathway narrows near it.

Fortunately, a thunderstorm can usually be anticipated by the formation of cumulonimbus clouds (Fig. 9.1). These are the towering anvil-shaped clouds that the God Thor was supposed to hit with his hammer to produce thunder. Today we know it merely represents the arrival of the cold fronts we see on the television weather map. There are turbulent currents within the thunderstorm that cause small ice particles to rise in the air currents while larger ice crystals brush past them to lower levels. This causes a transfer of electrons, making the top of the cloud positively charged and the bottom of the cloud negatively charged. The progress of a thunderstorm can be gauged by counting the number of seconds between a lightning flash and its corresponding clap of thunder. As sound travels a mile (1.6 km) in 5 seconds, the proximity of the storm's centre can be gauged. It is wise to seek shelter in a building or hard-roofed motor car. Soft-topped cars should be avoided. Ambulances may be at increased risk due to the induction effects of the vehicle radio aerial. During a storm strikes tend to be concentrated on high ground or tall buildings, where the distance between the ground and the thunder clouds is less so the resistance is less.

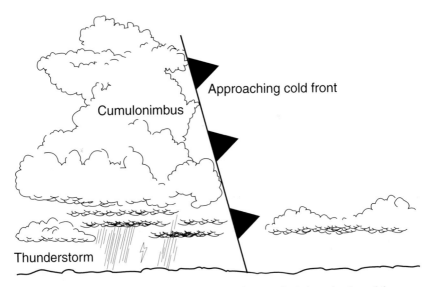

Figure 9.1   The relationship between a cold front, the cumulonimbus clouds and the thunderstorm.

Once the lightning has struck the ground there is a temporary reduction in electromotive force and so the risk of lightning strikes is reduced around the high spot. Provided you are at least 3 metres from the object that is the 'lightning conductor', to avoid the 'splash' of current around a strike, you will be relatively protected for an area equivalent to the height of the object. In other words, for a 30 metre building the safe zone is from 3 metres to 30 metres from the building in the shape of a cone drawn around the highest point (see Fig. 9.2).

Do not shelter under trees because of the splash, and do not carry anything that will act as a lightning conductor such as stretcher poles or scoop stretchers. Do not enter water, and avoid entering caves unless you have 3 metres head clearance and 1 metre to either side. Do not stand in gullies. Both caves and gullies act as natural discharge routes for lightning.

If you are part of a group you should separate to reduce the likelihood of a multiple strike. If caught out in the open, sit on a rucksack or other insulating material with your feet close to your buttocks. This will present as small an area as possible to current dissipating through the ground below you. If rescue attempts in open ground are necessary, you should crawl along the ground.

NATIONAL GRID POWER LINES

To enable efficient distribution of electricity around the country National Grid pylons carry voltages between 132 and 400 kilovolts. It cannot be con-

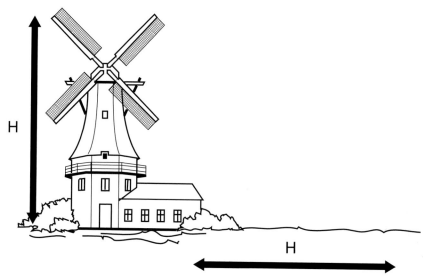

Figure 9.2 Safe zone around a tall structure during a thunderstorm.

sidered safe to get within 18 metres (20 yards) of a cable (Fig. 9.3). An accident involving power lines may well have caused automatic safety relays to operate, but this can occur as the result of bird strikes and the line may be re-energised at any moment. You must ensure the police confirm that the power has been fully discharged before you attempt a rescue.

The transmission lines feed grid supply points. These reduce the voltage to around 33 kilovolts. These are then fed to intermediate substations where the power is further reduced to 11 kilovolts. This is then fed via secondary distribution lines to distribution substations where the voltage is reduced to its final level of 415 and 240 volts. The voltage is changed by the means of transformers – these reduce the voltage but cause a corresponding increase in current availability.

DIRECT CURRENT, CIRCUITS, FUSES AND CAPACITORS

Electrical discharges from lightning are a one-way flow of electrons. This simple flow from negative to positive is known as direct current, and it is the type of power supply found in batteries. The simple electrical circuit is that of a wire starting from the negative pole of a battery, going via a switch to a load such as a motor or lamp, and then returning to the positive pole of the battery (Fig. 9.4).

For safety circuits are often fitted with a fuse. This is a wire that becomes hot when current flows through it. Excessive current for any reason will cause the fuse to melt, and thus the circuit is broken. Excessive current can

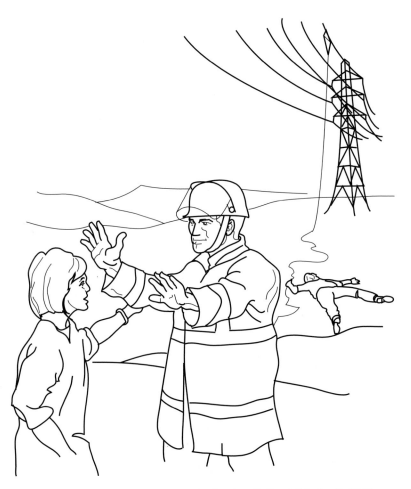

Figure 9.3   Applying the 1–2–3 of safety to a National Grid line incident.

flow if for any reason the load is bypassed and the current is able to flow more easily, as occurs in a short circuit. Fuses are unpredictable, however, as they do not always blow if there is a short circuit and yet they can blow due to age. Because changing fuses is a task many home-owner's fear, and to increase safety, many homes are now fitted with overload trip switches. These fit in the domestic fuse box but can be reset simply by pushing a button.

A capacitor is a simple electronic device. Simplistically this is two plates, one attached to the positive terminal of the power source and the other attached to the negative terminal. The plates are so close together that the positive charge attracts the negative charge, and so both are held on the plate. If you charge a capacitor, disconnect it from the power source and

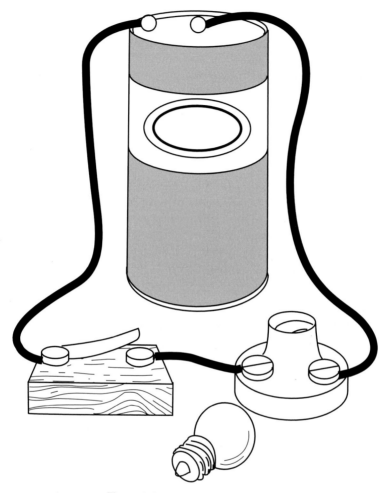

Figure 9.4 A simple electrical circuit.

touch the ends, you will receive a shock. A basic defibrillator consists of a battery, a capacitor, and the paddles and switch. Capacitors are used in many devices with motors, as their ability to charge and discharge can smooth an electric current and reduce the radio transmission effect of sparks. When used in these circumstances they are known as suppressors. Large capacitors can carry a charge capable of electrocution for many hours after the power has been disconnected. This is the reason for connecting the circuit to earth before making contact with it. The electrons held on the plate are attracted to the most favourable route.

A major disadvantage of direct current is that it cannot be readily stepped up and down in voltage, as is required for national distribution.

ALTERNATING CURRENT AND TRANSFORMERS

With alternating current the voltage across the power source starts at zero, increases to a maximum and decreases back to zero. The polarity of the contacts then reverses and the wave of power repeats. The cyclical wave pattern of power is repeated 50 times a second. This 50 hertz frequency often makes electrical apparatus hum, particularly when there is a transformer in the circuit. It can be 'transformed' into a different voltage because the electromagnetic effect of a coil of wire 'induces' a current to flow in a similar coil next to it. The number of turns in each coil determines the ratio of reduction.

It is important to remember that distribution substations in a domestic area might not have electrocuted someone with 240 or even 415 volts. They may have received 11 000 volts. The handling is completely different. Even with 415 volts a pair of regulation insulating rubber gloves and dry firefighter boots will prevent electrocution, but the insulation afforded by this level of protection is totally inadequate for 11 000 volts.

Three-phase supply

Power from the distribution substation is supplied via four wires. There are three-phase wires and a neutral wire that is physically earthed at the substation. The electromotive force between the consecutive phase wires is 415 volts, but between a phase wire and the neutral wire there is only 240 volts. Small buildings such as domestic homes are supplied with one of the phase wires and a neutral. This is called a single-phase supply. The phase wires are used in rotation to distribute the load so that each one serves every third building. In larger buildings it is more satisfactory to bring all four wires into the building. This is known as a three-phase supply. The load is then distributed equally between the phases by serving different areas of the building.

Fuses revisited

In early electrical installations both ends of the circuit had fuses installed. This system is no longer used because if the fuse on the neutral side of a circuit blew due to age or a fault, then the apparatus would not operate but would remain live and would feed to earth through anyone touching the apparatus. It is therefore important that the fuse is fitted on the live phase, rather than on the neutral side. Switches also must be fitted on the live phase side of the circuit.

Fuses can be inappropriately fitted, or if fitted correctly can be replaced with materials that do not fuse at the correct current. In particular sometimes the company fuse is replaced with a nail or a coin. This can create a great risk of fire or electrocution. You cannot be certain that a current will not flow because the switch is turned off or the fuse has blown. It is possible to buy from electronic shops such as Maplin and Tandy pen-sized electrical potential detectors. These are valuable devices for those likely to encounter dangerous circuits.

KEY POINT

- Insulation is only relative. If the voltage is great enough, any insulator will fail.

Self-test questions for Chapter 9

1. Give two circumstances where static electricity could be lethal.

2. A thunderclap occurs seven and a half seconds after a lightning flash. How far away is the storm?

3. What is the 'splash zone' around a lightning conductor?

4. What is the safe distance from a downed National Grid pylon cable?

5. What are the three voltages found in a distribution substation?

6. How does a fuse work?

7. Why is alternating current used by electricity companies?

Answers on p. 209.

Rail safety

BASIC PRINCIPLES

Railway safety requires a little knowledge and a lot of common sense. You should not enter the vicinity of the rails ('going trackside') without the knowledge of your control, who will inform Railtrack and the transport police. If you do go trackside then you need to know some basic terminology and safety principles (Fig. 10.1). The recognised position of safety is to stand in the cess. This is the space to either side of the tracks, clear of the ballast. The running rails are separated by a 4-foot gap (~1.2 metres) called the 4-foot way. Between adjacent tracks there is a 6-foot gap or way. Between pairs of tracks there may be a 10-foot way. Do not go on or near any line or cross the rails (except at a level crossing) unless it is absolutely necessary. Follow the route as instructed. Wherever possible use approved places of access to the lineside.

Make sure you know the permissible speed of trains and the direction they travel, unless look-out protection is provided. Trains normally drive

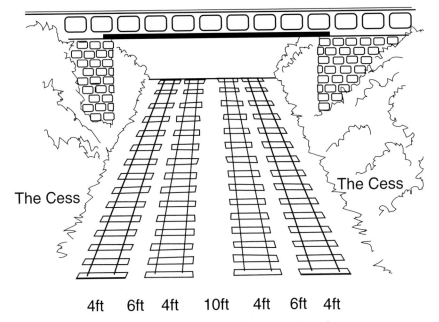

The Cess

The Cess

4ft   6ft   4ft   10ft   4ft   6ft   4ft

Figure 10.1   The terms applied to areas of the railway.

on the left, as on the roads, but if a line is being repaired trains may run in either direction on the remaining line. You must wear your high-visibility (HV) clothing – this must be clean and worn correctly. During darkness or when in a tunnel, you must wear high-visibility clothing with reflective markings. If necessary, you must wear a HV vest with reflective markings on top of other non-reflective clothing.

Be alert for approaching trains at all times – a signal at danger or raised level crossing barriers do not prevent the approach of a train. Trains may miss signals and electric trains can coast a considerable distance even when the power is off. The old semaphore signals are representations of a barrier. When horizontal they are at 'stop' and when raised they are at 'go'. The newer light signals are now almost universal. They have four alternatives. The red light means there is a train in the next section. One orange light indicates the next section is clear but there is a train in the section beyond. Two orange lights mean the next two sections are clear. Green means the track is clear for at least three sections.

Do not allow yourself to be distracted, for example by rendering first aid or using a radio when it is necessary to be alert for your own safety. It is particularly important to take extra care if wearing a hood because of weather conditions. Face the direction from which trains normally approach but beware of trains approaching from either direction. Where possible keep to the cess, and in particular avoid being on or between any lines. Take extra care in noisy areas, during high winds, darkness or poor visibility. You should remember that low sunlight glare can affect your visibility.

When possible cross the line by bridge or subway – if neither is available use a foot crossing and obey any warning signs. Look both ways before crossing the line or from one line to another. Step over, not on, rails because if there is a piece of metal on the track ahead the current from an electrified rail could be conducted to the running rails. Similarly do not walk on sleepers but walk on the ballast (the stone chippings). Sleepers are soaked in oil to preserve them and they can be slippery, especially in hot weather, when they 'sweat'. Equally in cold weather they rapidly ice up. Do not step between the blades of points as remote operation could cause movement that would trap your foot. They are operated at pressure of 60 pounds per square inch (~400 kilopascals), and can work even when the traction current is switched off. If you see an approaching train, move to the cess and signal to the driver that you have seen him by raising an arm in the air. Before the train passes, lower to the ground any equipment you are carrying. Remain in your position of safety until the train has passed and you can see no train is approaching, especially on another line. Avoid crossing in front of any moving train or vehicle, unless absolutely necessary, and do not go under any stationary vehicle or cross within 50 feet (or 15 metres) of stationary vehicles, unless you are sure they will not move.

POSITION OF SAFETY

This is a place that allows a clearance of at least the following distance between you (and anything you are wearing or carrying) and the nearest rail of any line on which a train is approaching:

- 6 feet 6 inches (or 2 metres) where permissible speed is over 100 mph (over 163 kilometres per hour);
- 4 feet (or 1.25 metres) where permissible speed is 100 mph or less.

Trains travelling at high speed, and even certain types of freight train at lesser speed, can create a draught as they pass that could cause you to lose your balance.

Even when you are in a position of safety, but close to the minimum clearance and it is not possible to move further away, take the following precautions:

1. Stand still, facing the line with your feet apart and make sure you have a firm footing.
2. Ensure your clothing is not loose and likely to flap.
3. Steady yourself against a structure or hold on to any secure object nearby.

4. If in a refuge or recess, use any handrail provided.
5. If standing against a wall, stand with your feet apart and with your back firmly against the wall. If necessary, lie down.
6. If you hear a train approach, do not assume it is on the normal line. Check which line it is running on.
7. If you are caught in the 6-foot or 10-foot way, with a train approaching from both directions and unable to reach a position of safety, then lie down immediately at a point where the ground is not obstructed. Never lie in the 4-foot way.

Limited clearances

Care must be taken when there is a limited clearance between the line on which trains may approach and other lines or adjacent structures. These are indicated by red and white chequered signs. When you move clear of an approaching train avoid standing where there is limited clearance. When walking past structures make sure your exit is clear. The blue and white chequered signs are provided only on lines where the permissible speed is over 100 mph. These indicate that adequate clearances or refuges exist only on the opposite side of the line. Use refuges or handholds while trains pass.

Tunnels

Do not enter a tunnel unless you are familiar with it or accompanied by a responsible member of Railtrack. Use a hand lamp. Make sure you know the location of the refuges and the clearances available. If a train approaches and you are unable to get to a refuge, lie down in the 6-foot way or between the line and the tunnel wall – whichever is safer – but never in the 4-foot way.

Converging lines

Take care there is sufficient clearance for your safety when alongside vehicles where lines converge. Do not ride on the step of a locomotive or vehicle.

Getting on or off moving engines, carriages and track appliances

Modern carriages have door control systems that prevent passengers alighting while the train is still in motion. Railway staff have the ability to circumvent the door systems but the principle must remain that you should not get on or off a moving vehicle.

Track maintenance machines

These can be noisy when working and could mask your hearing an approaching train. Take extra care and do not stand on the adjacent line to watch the machine working.

WARNING SYSTEMS

Detonators

These are small explosive charges placed on the rails to give audible warnings of danger ahead (Fig. 10.2). They are placed on the top of a running rail and secured by moulding the lead clips around the sides of the rail. In three- and four-rail systems they are fastened to the running rail furthest from the electrified rail. As the trains wheels pass over them, they explode, providing an audible warning to the driver. Detonators are found in sealed boxes in the front and rear cabs of trains, at stations and at depots. They are stored in a red metal container marked 'explosives'. Each detonator is colour coded and date stamped to show the year of manufacture. They should not be used in tunnels. When they are exploded, pieces of metal may fly long distances. Stand at least 30 yards (or 27 metres) away with your back to the detonators if trains pass.

Train-operated warning systems (TOWS)

This is an automatic system that give either a **safe** sound at 2- to 7-second intervals (to confirm its operation) or a **continuous** warning noise if a train is approaching. It is switched on and off by Railtrack personnel.

Track circuit operating clip

Automatic signals detect trains by the fact they connect the two running rails together. If a connection is made between the rails the automatic

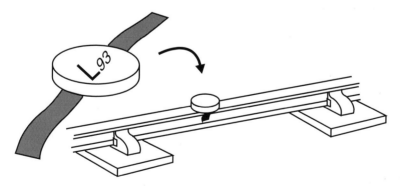

Figure 10.2 A track detonator.

signals will assume that there is a train in the section and automatically put the signals to danger. A track circuit operating clip is carried on every train and is exactly 4 feet long to prevent accidental connection to the third rail. The clip should always be first applied to the running rail furthest from the conductor rail.

ENGINE AND ROLLING STOCK CONSIDERATIONS

Old railway carriages were built as a wooden superstructure on flat-bed rolling stock. They were often insulated with asbestos. This has implications when they are involved in accidents, as they are both more liable to break up and when in this condition can present a health hazard. There is a policy of replacing old rolling stock and it may be expected that these carriages are now rare. New carriages have pneumatically operated doors that can be operated by the external door-operating switch. Access to the driver's cab can be gained in the same way.

Before rescue work is started on a carriage the pantograph, if present, must be in the lowered position and the battery-isolating switch should be turned to off. In some of the old electrical traction units the capacitor can contain polychlorinated biphenyls. These are being replaced but are exceptionally dangerous in the presence of fire and water. Full chemical protection suits should therefore be worn by fire personnel dealing with such a fire, and the situation dealt with as if it were a chemical incident.

Hazards such as asbestos in carriages was an issue that British Rail were aware of and could rapidly advise the emergency services about once the identification number of the rolling stock involved was known. Recent attempts to gain up-to-date information suggest that immediate access to this information has now been complicated by privatisation.

ELECTRIFIED LINES

Overhead system

The overhead power system supplies electricity to engine units through lines electrified at up to 25 000 volts (Fig. 10.3). The pylons themselves are not electrified but all lines suspended from them must be considered so. Not only is there danger from contact with these wires, but the current is also sufficiently great to arc across short distances, particularly in damp weather. Where possible, walk at track level, on normal roadways, station platforms, etc.

Always regard the overhead line equipment and its attachments as live. Keep yourself and your clothing, tools and equipment at least 9 feet (or 2.75 metres) from:

● anything attached to or hanging from the overhead equipment;

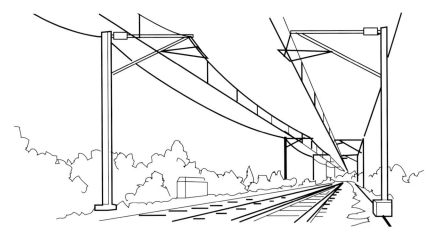

Figure 10.3 Overhead line equipment.

- any broken or displaced wire connected to the overhead line;
- equipment, whether hanging or lying on the ground.

Take extra care on embankments, structures or vehicles that could bring you within that distance. Carry long articles horizontally – take extra care with pipes, rods, poles, etc. Get someone to help you if necessary.

KEY POINT

- Do not carry out any work requiring any part of your body, or any tool or materials you are using, to approach nearer than 9 feet (or 2.75 metres) to the live equipment from any direction.

DO NOT WORK ABOVE LIVE OVERHEAD LINE EQUIPMENT.

Conductor rail system (Fig 10.4)

These lines have a raised third rail (the conductor rail) supported on insulators fixed to the sleepers. The conductor rail is electrified at up to 750 volts. In some areas a raised fourth rail is also provided – regard this in the same way as the conductor rail.

KEY POINT

- Always regard the conductor rail and its connections as live.

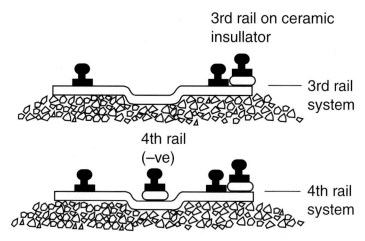

Figure 10.4 Cross-section of the electrified rail system.

The following safety points apply to conductor rail systems.

- Avoid crossing conductor rails unless absolutely necessary. If you have to cross, do so at a gap or where protective boarding is provided.
- Do not step on, touch or allow your clothing, tools or equipment to touch a conductor rail or its connections.
- Do not step on protection boarding or between a conductor rail and the adjacent running rail – step over both in one movement.
- Do not touch the collector shoes or their connections on any electric train or locomotive, whether or not they are in contact with the conductor rail.
- Do not step into flood water that may be in contact with the conductor rail.

ACTION IN AN EMERGENCY

Protection of the line

If an emergency occurs that could endanger trains, immediate action must be taken to stop trains and clear the obstruction. Do not endanger yourself. The signal operator may be able to stop trains – make contact and explain what has happened. Make use of any lineside telephone to contact the signal operator or control point. If you need the power to be cut off it is important to give a power pylon reference number for the power station to identify which section is to be isolated. Similarly for the signals to be correctly set the signal box will need to know a signal number. While sections can be identified from either number, it is faster to give the right number to the right control.

You may consider improvising a track circuit operating clip, but if you do so you must be very careful to make sure you do not touch any electrified rail. You may also consider short circuiting the power rail in a dire emergency. This must obviously be done in such a manner as to avoid electrocution. It is not uncommon for wild animals to cause a short circuit and power control centres will often attempt to re-energise the track before investigating the cause. While it is a useful way of rapidly alerting the rail authorities to an emergency, it cannot be regarded as a definite confirmation of safety. When electric trains lose traction current they will try to coast to the next electrified section unless there is a signal against them. On a down gradient they may travel several miles in this way.

If unable to contact the signal operator, proceed back along the line for 2 kilometres in the direction from which trains normally approach. If a train approaches show a red flag or raise your arms above the head. During darkness exhibit a red light or wave any light violently.

Making an emergency telephone call

The steps below should be followed when making an emergency call.

- State that is an **emergency** call.
- State who you are and give the exact location by using the identification number of a signal or overhead line equipment structure.
- State what has happened.
- Make sure your message has been understood.

Figure 10.5 shows signs that indicate the presence of a trackside emergency phone.

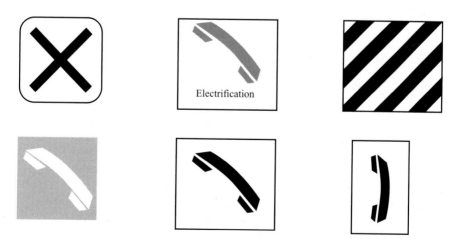

Figure 10.5   Signs indicating a trackside emergency telephone.

ELECTRIC SHOCK RESCUE

Electric shock from overhead traction equipment

If the casualty is not on the ground, do not attempt rescue unless you have the assistance and advice of a railway employee trained in first aid for electrical accidents. However you should immediately follow the procedure to get the electricity switched off.

If the casually is completely below live overhead line equipment and no part of the body is nearer than 3 feet (or 1 metre) from the live overhead line equipment, it is not essential for the electricity to be switched off. It is perfectly safe to touch the person since there is no harmful electric charge retained in the body.

You must make quite sure for your own safety that no part of your body, clothing, anything you are holding or the casualty gets within 3 feet (or 1 metre) of the live overhead line equipment or anything in contact with it.

KEY POINT

- If the casualty is not completely below, or is within 3 feet (or 1 metre) of live overhead line equipment, it is essential that the electricity is switched off before the casualty is approached or touched.

Electric shock from conductor rails

If the casualty is touching a conductor rail the electricity should, if at all possible, be switched off before you touch the casualty. Railtrack staff may carry a pole for shorting the third rail. This causes the overload trip to activate at the power control centre. However, this can occur when an animal encounters the third rail and staff tend routinely to reconnect the power. It is only if the trip activates repeatedly that the control centre will investigate.

If it is not possible to have the electricity switched off immediately, take the following precautions before you touch the casualty.

- Cover your hands with something that will not conduct electricity. A dry mackintosh or an article of dry clothing or rubber gloves will do.
- Wet articles are unsafe if moisture on the surface makes contact with wet clothing or skin.
- Stand on dry non-conducting material, such as a mackintosh, wood, thick carpet, thick newspaper, glass or rubber. If none of these is available, move the casualty clear with a dry rope or a dry wooden pole. Do not use anything made of metal.

Electric shock from other circuits

If the casualty is touching a live conductor, switch off the electricity before you touch the casualty if the switch is near. If you know the voltage is not above 750 volts and you cannot readily switch it off, follow the instructions as for the conductor rails. If you are unsure of the voltage, do not approach the casualty until you are assured the power is off.

THE LONDON UNDERGROUND

The London Underground system has been travelled on by millions of people, and its famous map is printed in countless different documents. Technically there are ten lines, but for historical reasons there are only eight line controllers. The line controllers are responsible for the safe and efficient running of the railway. They rely on information from railway staff, particularly signal operators, and computerised information to help them manage any situation. They have a wide range of communication and control systems at their disposal and they are the only people who can confirm that traction current has been discharged.

The Underground's telephone system

The London Underground operates its own telephone system. The emergency number that connects with the British Transport Police Information Room is, like the British Telecom system, 999.

London Underground signalling

The London Underground uses a simple signalling system with a green light to proceed and a red light for danger. Each signal has an identification number. The majority of signals are worked automatically by the passage of a train. These signals can be identified by the letter 'A' in front of the three-digit identification number. Signals at junctions are controlled by a signal operator and have an identification of one or two letters followed by one or two numbers.

Fully automatic signals will change from green to red as soon as the train passes it, and then revert to green again as soon as the train leaves that signalling section. Semi-automatic signals will turn to red as a train passes but will remain on red until manually reset in the signal box. Electric locks in the system prevent this from occurring if there is still a train in the signalling section.

At track level both types of signal are equipped with a 'trainstop'. This is a metal arm that moves up when the signal changes to red. If a train passes a raised trainstop, the metal arm knocks open a tripcock valve at the front of the train. Compressed air that is keeping the brakes off escapes from the system and the train is stopped.

Semi-automatic signals can be used to protect people on the track by placing collars over the reset lever in the signal box. This can be arranged by a station supervisor. Automatic signals provide no protection.

At locations on bends where there is insufficient sighting distance on a signal there will be a repeater signal. These differ in having a green and a yellow light. Green shows the signal ahead is on proceed, and yellow means the signal ahead is at red.

In depots and sidings rotating circular shunt signals can be found. They consist of a white disc with a red bar through the centre. The red bar represents a barrier in the same way as a semaphore signal. Horizontal means danger and diagonal means proceed. These signals are all semi-automatic.

Single- and double-track tunnels

The Bakerloo, Central, Jubilee, Piccadilly, Northern and Victoria lines all have single-track (tube) tunnels. The minimum space between the tunnel wall and the carriage is 9 inches (~23 centimetres; see Fig. 10.6). There is therefore insufficient room for persons to enter a tube tunnel while trains are running. The traction current must be discharged and the trains stopped before entry to the tunnel is made. The Underground system relies on the movement of trains to provide sufficient air changes on board for the needs of the passengers. In the rush hour people will start collapsing if trains are brought to a halt for more than 40 minutes. It is therefore imperative that rescues requiring the halting of trains are made expeditiously.

Double-track tunnels are to be found on the Circle, District, East London, Hammersmith & City and Metropolitan lines. The running rails are separated by a 6-foot way, but the overhang of the carriages reduces this to a 3-foot actual clearance. Again, the gap between the tunnel wall and the train can be as little as 9 inches (~23 cm). Under certain circumstances London Underground staff are allowed to work in double-track tunnels while trains continue to run; however, emergency service personnel should ensure that the traction current has been discharged before they enter the tunnel.

At stations the positive rail is usually furthest from the platform. There are some exceptions to this rule, and between stations the positive rail may be on either side.

Traction current

Electricity to the Underground is supplied from two power stations and is distributed to substations located along the line, where it is fed into the line in sections at 630 volts DC. Each section is isolated from the other by a

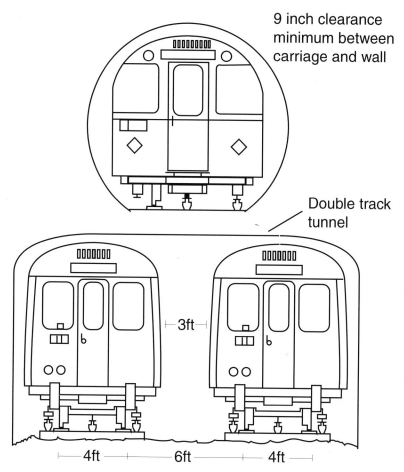

9 inch clearance minimum between carriage and wall

Double track tunnel

3ft

4ft — 6ft — 4ft

Figure 10.6   The layout of single and double track in London Underground tunnels.

physical break in the rail, called a rail gap. These are indicated by a tri-angular white plate with a red light at each corner. These lights are illumin-ated if the section ahead has the power turned off. The driver, on seeing these lights, will attempt to stop the train before it enters the dead section. If this cannot be done, the driver will continue into the section and attempt to coast to the next station. The driver must not stop the train over the gap as this will allow the traction current to pass from a live into a dead section.

Short circuit devices (SCDs)

There are various types of short circuit device that are designed for the use of Underground personnel. They consist of insulated metal bars that can connect between the positive and negative rails. They are placed on the rails in that order. The short circuit will operate relays that disconnect the power. It is then imperative that contact is made with the line controller by radio or telephone within 7 minutes or the line controller will attempt to restore the power to keep the service running. The line controller will attempt this three times. However, once the line controller has been contacted, traction current will not be restored until it has been confirmed it is safe to do so.

Telephones and plungers

At tunnel stations headwall telephones are to be found in black or brown boxes marked 'Private' or 'Tunnel Telephone'. Between stations there are further telephones that may be used to contact the line controller. Where there is a rail gap just ahead or to the rear of a platform there are boxes containing a plunger that will discharge the current. To operate the seal on the box is broken, the box opened and the plunger depressed for 3 seconds. The line controller needs to be contacted within 7 minutes.

The Victoria Line is the only one entirely below ground and is also the only fully automatic train. After opening and closing the doors the train operator simultaneously pushes two buttons. The train is then driven by codes, fed to it through the running rails. On the Victoria Line the headwall telephones have been replaced by headwall plungers. Also, along the length of the platform are located three code destroyers. These are yellow boxes containing a black paper disc with yellow arrows indicating where the disc is to be punctured. Operating a code destroyer will not discharge the traction current but will apply the emergency brakes to any train for 400 feet (120 metres) either side of the platform. Under certain circumstances the operator can still drive the train but is limited to 9 mph (14.4 kilometres per hour).

Detrainment of passengers

There are occasions when it becomes necessary to move people off a train even though it is not at a station. This process is the responsibility of the Underground staff, but since it only occurs in exceptional circumstances the emergency services may be involved. The easiest method is by direct transfer. This is where two trains are brought alongside each other and immobilised. The seat backs are then laid between the trains as a bridge and passengers decanted. Unfortunately only certain trains are now suitable for this type of transfer, as it requires seats without backs attached to the bases.

The alternative is to bring the trains alongside each other and immobilise them. The traction current is then discharged and ladders placed at the end of the trains. Passengers are then transferred a car at a time. Only when transfer methods cannot be used will the line controller authorise staff to walk passengers to the nearest station. Passengers are detrained in manageable groups, counted and escorted to the station.

'One under'

All London ambulance crews will be familiar with the phrase that indicates that a person has fallen or thrown themselves on to the track in front of an approaching Underground train. The Underground system has over 270 stations and around 100 people every year end up under a train. The average train is approximately 350 feet (106 metres) long and takes about 400 feet (120 metres) to stop when travelling at 35 mph (56 kph). Approximately 75% of people are trying to kill themselves, and around 40% succeed. About a quarter of casualties are able to crawl out with help. About one in five are held down, alive, and the train moved. In a smaller proportion, the train is removed to recover the body. In only one in every 20 cases does the train need to be jacked up.

Working under an Underground train has to be rapid, which suits the ambulance crews as the environment is both dirty and hot. Not only is the ambient temperature high, but almost everything that you touch is hot enough to burn, owing to the friction that is generated during the running of the train.

Escalator entrapment

Escalators have emergency stop buttons at both the top and the bottom of the staircase. If operated the machine will stop almost immediately. For this reason a warning should be shouted before operating the emergency button. Once an escalator has been stopped it cannot be restarted without the use of a key. If people are trapped in the combs it is possible to use apparatus to lift them. This is usually located in the newel post at either the top or the bottom of the staircase. Access to this equipment may only be gained by the use of a key. Great care must be taken when removing these tools as they could fall into the machine room. Before their use the escalator must be fully isolated, and normally the station supervisor will carry out the lifting procedure. This advice is specific to Underground station escalators, but also may apply to other escalators. In other places the lifting procedure should be delegated to the fire service.

KEY POINT

- Never go lineside without the track operator being aware of your presence.

Self-test questions for Chapter 10

1. What is the area to the side of the railway tracks known as?

2. What should you do when a train approaches?

3. What does a blue and white chequered sign on a tunnel mean?

4. What is the minimum distance to be kept from any electrified part of an overhead line equipment?

5. What is the voltage of the overhead electrification system?

6. What is the voltage of the conductor rail system?

7. What is the minimum distance to be kept from an overhead electrification system in order to rescue a casualty?

8. A casualty has fallen onto the conductor rail between Railtrack stations. What action should you take to retrieve the casualty?

9. What does a track circuit operating clip do?

10. What information is stamped on a railway detonator?

11. What is the minimum clearance between train and single (tube) tunnel wall?

12. How does a trainstop work?

13. Which London Underground line uses code destroyers?

Answers on p. 210.

11

Aircraft incidents

INTRODUCTION

There are many types of incident involving aircraft. Most of these incidents take place at an airport and are generally handled by the airport emergency services. If it is necessary to attend an airport to treat a casualty you should not use blue or green beacons when airside. If your vehicle is fitted with an amber beacon this may be used. You should contact air traffic control and follow a marshalling vehicle to the scene. Wear high-visibility clothing and you may need ear protectors.

However, from time to time these incidents develop into potential if not actual aircraft accidents, and help is sought from the external emergency services. In addition to this, a large proportion of aircraft accidents occur off airport.

As you may well be the first attending emergency personnel at one of these incidents, either on or off airport, it is essential that you are aware of the immediate needs in the early stages of such incidents, and in particular your role in satisfying these needs.

AIRCRAFT ACCIDENT TYPES

There are two types of aircraft accident; these are described in Box 11.1. The type of accident will influence the casualty outcome and the probable chances of survival for persons involved. Your speed of response to the incident and the effectiveness of your role on arrival will directly influence this in turn.

> **Box 11.1**   Types of aircraft accident
>
> *High-speed accident*
>
> This type of accident usually occurs during flight at altitude. An example of this was the Pan-Am Flight 101 that blew up over Lockerbie. Such an incident often results in the pilot not being in control, possibly due to mid-air collisions, loss of control functions or engine failure. These accidents are generally non-survivable.
>
> *Low-speed accident*
>
> This is an accident that usually occurs during landing or take-off, on approach to the runway, or immediately after the take-off on climb out. Alternatively the aircraft may already be on the ground and may have been involved with a ground vehicle or a building. In this scenario the pilot is more likely to be in control and the cabin staff able to direct staff and passengers. This type of incident is survivable.

AIRPORT AIRCRAFT INCIDENTS

There are a number of types of incident involving aircraft that can happen at an airport. Usually the response to an airport will be on declaration of a 'full emergency' or 'ground incident'. On these occasions you would normally respond to the airport emergency service rendezvous point (RVP) and await further instructions. Signposts to airports indicate RVP locations; these have yellow letters on a green background.

In the event of an 'aircraft accident imminent' call your response to the rendezvous point would be the same. However, in the event of an accident happening, you would be escorted to the accident scene, if at a different location from the RVP.

In the event of a major incident the airport fire service will not have enough personnel or equipment to resource firefighting and rescue for long periods, especially in the case of a large aircraft with up to 600 passengers.

First aid/casualty handling

Firefighters are instructed not be distracted from the first part of the life-saving role, that of rescue, as long as there are people trapped within an aircraft or there is a fire to be extinguished before rescue can take place.

Casualty clearances by the fire service purely relate to removal of trapped or injured persons from the aircraft to the casualty clearance zone.

OFF-AIRPORT INCIDENTS

Airport incidents have the advantage that a specialist fire service is immediately on hand to deal with any incident. In the event of an off-airport incident there could be a large external fire still burning or the fire may have done damage leaving a badly decomposed and charred wreck with bodies spread over a large area.

Foam will always be applied to the fuselage if it is still intact and to any area where persons may still be trapped and any area adjacent to where fire service personnel are likely to be working. It must be assumed that fumes will be present and also some carbon fibre composites may be involved. Any foam blanket must be topped-up from time to time throughout rescue operations. Foam covers both holes and obstructions on the ground, obscuring them from view, and acts as a medium on which to slip. Particular care must be taken when walking through foam.

An inner cordon will be established as soon as practicable. Always remember to preserve evidence or make a note of evidence that has to be altered or removed in the course of casualty extrication. Keep the numbers of personnel in the immediate crash site to a minimum.

HAZARDS ASSOCIATED WITH AIRCRAFT

Before charging into the unknown it is essential to have knowledge of the hazards associated with aircraft and how they can affect the process of achieving rescue goals at an aircraft accident.

On-airport hazards

Airports are inherently dangerous places where normal rules do not necessarily apply. For instance, you cannot simply put on your beacons and assume that aircraft will give way to you. You must never proceed onto an airport without establishing radio contact with airport air traffic control (AATC) or being escorted by a member of the airport operations team or the police. Never enter a live runway without permission. Airport authorities frequently specify that vehicles operating airside should have a level of insurance capable of covering the expense of damage to aircraft.

Aircraft engines

Be aware that when attending an aircraft incident on an airport other aircraft will possibly be operating, presenting a significant hazard to both health and equipment. Keep well away from these aircraft, in particular avoiding their engine intakes and exhausts. Never approach an aircraft with its engines running. Even standing at the side of an aircraft engine on 'tick over' can prove hazardous; it will pick you up from the site and 'liquidise' you.

Stay back from the engines at least to a distance of 8 metres. As a rule do not pass the line of the nose when approaching from the front and stay back at least 45 metres from the exhaust area when approaching from the rear. Remember that these distances apply also above and below the engines, so do not even think about approaching either over or under the mainplane (wing).

If an aircraft has crashed it is unlikely that its engines will still be running. However, there are many other incidents where an aircraft engine may be left on or other aircraft may still be operating around you.

Aircraft undercarriages

Brake and wheel assemblies on aircraft can overheat due to heavy braking on landing or long taxiing following landing. This often leads to smoking and in some cases visible flame. Approach to all undercarriage incidents must be fore and aft. The use of firefighting jets may result in rim failure and wheel fragmentation caused by spot cooling and uneven metal expansion.

All personnel and equipment must remain clear of an area stretching outward from the undercarriage in an ever-widening fan shape at an angle of approximately 45° either side from the centre of the assembly.

Fuel

There are, broadly speaking, two categories of aviation fuel:

- gasoline – known as Avgas;
- kerosene – known as Avtur, Avtag or Avcat. It may also be called JP 1, 4 or 5, or ATK, ATG or ATC.

Avgas is used in piston engine aircraft including all the older propeller-driven aircraft and a large proportion of light prop aircraft in general use today. It is supplied in three grades. Each has a flashpoint of –40°C and has a rapid flame spread rate of 200–250 metres per minute.

Kerosene fuels are turbine fuels and are used in all jetprop, turbojet, turbofan and propfan engines. Avtag has similar properties to gasoline, but the others have higher flame points and much lower flame spread rates.

These are obviously very flammable liquids, but can also be toxic if absorbed through the skin or inhaled in concentration.

Aircraft construction and materials

Wreckage from aircraft accidents contains a wide range of materials that are potentially hazardous. Individuals risk being exposed to these materials in high concentrations for a short duration or a combination of levels over protracted periods. The precise identification of these materials is difficult, given the nature of aircraft accidents.

Mechanical hazards

All aircraft will present some form of mechanical hazard to rescue personnel during operations at an aircraft accident. The fluids, gases and pneumatics in pressurised systems present hazards owing to stored energy as well as the inherent problems of contact with the system contents. Electrical systems and batteries may be live for some time in badly damaged aircraft. Control systems may also be operable and can be spring-loaded or weight-balanced, presenting unexpected hazards. There is the more obvious problem of working in areas that may be unstable and have sharp and jagged structures, as well as the ever-present risk of fire.

Metals and oxides

Fire-damaged aircraft structures will contain an unknown variety and quantity of metals and oxides within the wreckage remains. Aluminium and aluminium oxides will be present as structural materials in significant quantities and, where fire has occurred, in variable particle sizes. Aluminium is also alloyed with magnesium, zinc, copper, titanium, lithium, zirconium, chromium, boron and beryllium.

Radioactive materials

Radioactive materials are known to have been used in some components, although specific activities, quantities and incidence of use are very low. If the presence of radioactive materials is suspected, seek advice from the fire officer.

Thorium has been used in the past as an alloy with magnesium in castings of some engine intakes, compressors and accessory gearboxes. Although apparently discontinued, it is likely that such components may remain in use for some years to come.

Depleted uranium has also been known to be used in early versions of B747 (jumbo) aircraft. Titanium is used in gaseous tritium light sources generally to mark emergency exits.

Composites

Composite materials are used in many aircraft structures and components, and in various applications. The dust and fibres produced by many of the materials when damaged are known to produce nuisance hazards and may produce chronic health conditions affecting the respiratory system and the eyes. Long-term damage may result to body tissue and particles could enter the bloodstream through open wounds, and even through the skin, with serious consequences to health. When sufficient quantities of fibre dust become airborne, breathing difficulties can be experienced. Full protective clothing must be worn including breathing apparatus when fighting fires where these components are known or suspected of being involved. However, for prolonged operations in the area contaminated by composite wreckage, it is recommended that chemical protection suits be worn. Disposal of composite materials should be as for asbestos.

Carbon fibre composites and manufactured mineral fibres are known to be conductive. Consideration should be given to warning any operator of electrical or electronic equipment downwind of any accident involving large amounts of these products with a view to closing down until any particle cloud has passed.

Normal chemical incident procedures should be invoked for the purposes of restriction of personnel in affected areas and decontamination. Helicopters must not be allowed over the affected area. The downdraught from these aircraft will disturb any foam blanket and agitate the carbon fibres, lifting and spreading them into the atmosphere.

MILITARY AIRCRAFT

Additional hazards are directly associated with military aircraft, as listed in Box 11.2. Military aircraft will normally carry the standard danger, warning and direction markings for escape systems or other aircraft systems that can give visual indication to firefighting crews of the hazards that may be present.

Radar/radiation hazard

While civilian aircraft use radar, it is normally only used for weather indication and is of small size and power output. Military radar application will be of a greater extent with the possibility of large power output when switched on and in the search mode. Aircraft such as the Nimrod and the AWACS utilise radar to search over large areas at very long range in order to detect aircraft or vessels, and can represent a significant hazard when operating. There may be long-term medical implications for personnel exposed to a high-power radar signal.

Box 11.2 Hazards associated with military aircraft

Radar
Infrared laser sights
Weapons systems
Pyrotechnics
Aircrew escape systems
 MDC (miniature detonating cord)
 LCC (linear cutting cord)
 Canopy jettison
Cargo and equipment

Infrared laser sights

Increasingly, a number of fighter aircraft are fitted with an infrared laser guidance system for weapons targeting. These systems usually operate from the nose area of the aircraft and fire through clear glass panels. The signal emitting from these systems can damage delicate eye tissue and all personnel should be aware that they should not look directly into these glass panels unless it has been confirmed that the guidance system is inoperative.

Weapons systems

The weapons systems employed on military aircraft are too numerous for each one to be covered individually; however, they may be outlined and grouped as:

- missiles for attack or defence;
- missiles ICBM (Tomahawk, etc.)
- torpedoes;
- bombs, cannon, machine gun, etc.

While these weapons differ in size and use, they may all represent a hazard when involved with fire. It is unlikely that a weapon would explode instantaneously when affected by fire, because the way it reacts is subject to many variables. For example, the rate at which a weapon absorbs heat is dependent on the thermal density of the material used as the explosive. The main charge may not be as sensitive as the inner detonator charge, and may provide some insulation. The size and density of the external weapon casing may delay detonation, by providing an insulation barrier to the effects of heat. Though the obvious danger from the weapon is from the high explosive, it should also be remembered that on missile systems the weapon is propelled by specialist rocket fuels and oxidisers; when heated these may react before the explosive. Thus rockets can ignite and propel themselves out of control in a military aircraft fire. Aircraft also frequently have chaff ejectors that discharge a mass of metal chaff to the rear and side of the aircraft to confuse and divert anti-aircraft missiles.

Pyrotechnics

These substances take many forms, and some may contain small explosive or detonation devices. They range from signal cartridges and distress flares to the large marker and detection device used in maritime reconnaissance.

These types of device are designed in such a way and stored or used in such a specialist application that they would not normally represent a significant hazard, nor detonate en masse, when involved in fire.

Aircrew escape systems

These are systems that form part of the aircraft or are fitted into the aircraft in order to facilitate the protection of aircrew in an emergency. Their very operation is of an explosive nature and can represent a potential hazard to firefighters, if handled incorrectly.

The ejector seat and canopy systems fitted to fighter and some trainer aircraft form a joint escape system. The escape system is arranged so that on the initiation of an eject sequence, the canopy system operates first through one of three systems:

1. *MDC (miniature detonation cords)*. This is arranged around and through the overhead of the canopy transparency and explodes, shattering the material, to allow the pilot and ejector seat to pass through safely (Fig. 11.1).
2. *LCC (linear cutting cords)*. This system is similar in concept to MDC, but is arranged around the periphery of the canopy frame and is designed to separate the transparency from the frame and allow the airflow to carry it clear.
3. *Canopy jettison*. This system utilises rocket packs, fitted to the canopy frame, which when activated, fire and carry the full canopy and frame clear of the aircraft (usually to the rear).

Ejector seats

The modern ejector seat (Fig. 11.2) has changed greatly from its early counterpart. In most cases, to safely effect rescue, it requires only one seat safety pin to be inserted into the seat pan firing handle. With this mechanism made safe, the other parts of the seat system cannot operate due to sequenc-

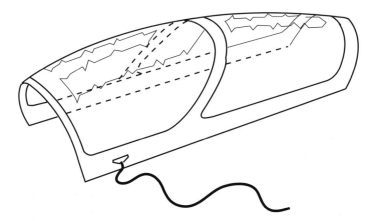

Figure 11.1   Aircraft canopy with miniature detonator cord exposed.

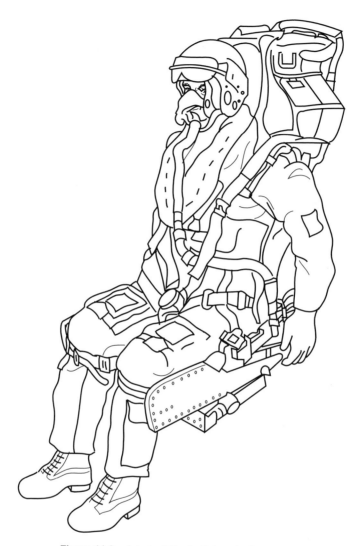

Figure 11.2 A typical Martin Baker ejector seat.

ing; however, it should be remembered that they could be activated if the relevant pin is withdrawn accidentally.

The harness arrangements on ejector seats vary from type to type, and it is not possible to cover fully all the arrangements in this manual. Generally they are of the 'five-point' type with a central release bar, and additional releases for dinghy, personal equipment connector (PEC) and leg restraint. The best course of action is, through training, to become familiar with the types that you are likely to encounter.

Cargo and equipment hazards

The type and amount of cargo and specialist equipment carried on a military transport aircraft will be dependent on its role or mission requirement and can include such things as small arms, specialist fuels, toxic or radioactive materials, vehicles, etc.

RESCUE TACTICS FOR HELICOPTERS

Approach to an accident/fire situation should be as for conventional aircraft but personnel must be aware of the hazards associated with main and tail rotors. Where these are still turning, great care should be taken when moving towards the fuselage.

Under crash conditions, it is advisable to approach the helicopter in a crouching position if the main rotor is still turning. The rotor blades will continue to turn and sag lower even if the engine has stopped. It must be assumed that these will sag below head level.

Never approach or position appliances and personnel to the front or rear of crashed military helicopters, as there is always a danger of missiles being released.

Where water-actuated devices are fitted into the wheel hubs, care must be taken not to stand directly at the side of the wheels in case the disc covering the device blows off. This could cause serious injury to nearby persons. A direct jet of water could activate the device. Approach the helicopter from the downhill side if possible.

KEY POINT

- An aircraft incident is a complex chemical hazard as well as a crash site.

Self-test questions for Chapter 11

1. You are instructed to attend a full emergency at your local airport. Where do you go and what identifies where it is?

2. An accident has occurred to a workman on the taxi routes of a small provincial airfield. What actions do you take on arrival at the main gate?

3. What is the minimum distance to keep away from an aircraft engine?

4. Give two reasons for using a foam blanket at an aircraft fire.

5. What is a major problem of using a foam blanket?

6. What is MDC, and what does it do?

7. What influences the selection of a casualty clearing point at an airfield crash site?

Answers on p. 211.

Rescue in confined spaces/collapsed structures

TYPICAL INCIDENTS

Rescue of casualties from confined spaces may be due to the casualties actively seeking to occupy a space and then finding themselves trapped, as in a pot-holing accident. Alternatively, it may be by their accidental introduction into the environment, as in falling down a disused mine shaft. Most commonly, however, it is by a building or structure that normally would not cause confinement being distorted around them. Examples of these are:

- Moorgate tube disaster
- Putney flats explosion
- Armenian earthquake
- Peak cavern incident
- Abbeystead disaster
- Whitworth gas explosion
- Aberfan disaster
- Brighton bombing.

These situations provide examples of both actual and relative entrapment and are classic situations where immediate care saves lives. This, however, results in the paramedic or immediate care doctor working in conditions that can pose considerable hazards. The Lancashire Fire and Rescue Service 'Safety at Scene' course has a practical session on rescue from confined spaces. It employs a training gallery at the Fire Training Centre that allows for the rapid extrication of rescuers who cannot cope with the environment.

This is far preferable to the rescuer only realising the blind panic of their claustrophobia when in a real-life situation. Rescuers who could be faced with the challenges of this type of environment should make arrangements to attend the course or have similar training at a local fire service training establishment.

HAZARDS

Irrespirable atmospheres

Oxygen deficiency (or surplus)

In a confined space the concentration of oxygen may be reduced by displacement with other gases, or by consumption if there are casualties, animals or fire. The oxygen concentration may rise if oxygen administration equipment is used in a confined space. Using high-flow oxygen effectively puts 3 gallons of pure oxygen into a space every minute. It does not take many minutes before the concentration of oxygen will have risen to the point where minor smouldering or sparking could cause you and your casualty to ignite spontaneously. Lighting equipment introduced into the area should be intrinsically safe. Forced ventilation must be considered in any confined space where casualties are to be found. This can be either by using compressed air to displace the foul air, or by using air-extraction systems. The advantage of using compressed air is that pure air is taken into the environment, but the air must be introduced at the bottom of the confined space to ensure that the heavier carbon dioxide is displaced. The mere introduction of oxygen into the area will not reduce the level of carbon dioxide, which is a potent stimulant to respiration.

Carbon dioxide

Carbon dioxide is a gas heavier than air and will tend to accumulate in basements and cellars, particularly when there is respiration in progress. The respiratory activity of plant material, such as silage, grain and brewery yeast, is frequently unrecognised as a cause of an irrespirable atmosphere.

Carbon monoxide

Carbon monoxide is produced by inadequate combustion of carbon fuel. It may be due to internal combustion engines or due to badly ventilated gas or charcoal fires. It can escape from damaged flues and chimneys. It has no describable odour and is poisonous due to its great affinity for haemoglobin, binding to the molecule preferentially to oxygen. People experienced in working with carbon monoxide can often detect its presence, but for many headache, nausea and confusion are the only signs that unconsciousness will soon follow. Immediate treatment is with high-concentration oxygen. Those with neurological signs need hyperbaric oxygen at the nearest facility. The gas is flammable and can be explosive.

Sewer gases

These gases, produced by rotting vegetation, comprise a variable combination of hydrogen sulphide, methane, sulphur dioxide and trichloroethylene. These can be poisonous, do not support respiration, and are flammable and explosive. In 1985 a group of people visited the Abbeystead pumping station in Lancashire. Rotting vegetation had caused an accumulation of methane in the structure, which was not normally open to the public. It is believed that a cigarette triggered an explosion that demolished the pumping station and caused many fatalities.

Domestic hazards

Mains services

Although the collapse of a building will usually cause the electricity company's main fuse to blow and render the wiring safe, this cannot be assumed. Care must be taken therefore around wires and cables, as well as near domestic appliances that may be live.

Household chemicals

Containers of household chemicals may have ruptured, releasing strong detergents, caustic preparations and solvents. Together with compressed gas cannisters, these can pose a serious risk.

Fire

Fire may be present as a result of the overturning of sources of flame, spillages of flammable liquids onto hot surfaces, etc. The building may be lying like a loosely stacked bonfire – not an ideal environment to find yourself having to crawl carefully through. If fire may have to be fought when penetrating a collapsed building, the need to take a hose needs to be considered. The use of large quantities of water could precipitate further collapse, cause flooding, and even pressurisation of the hose could apply pressure to vulnerable supporting structures.

Flooding

The disruption of water mains, drains and sewers can all precipitate flooding of subterranean areas. In caves, pot-holes and mines flooding may have been the event that precipitated entrapment. The rescue is then very dependent on the ability to control the entry of water into the underground system, and failing that, on the weather itself.

Hypothermia

Immobility in a cold damp environment where the body is making a large area of contact with the ground allows heat loss to such a degree that hypothermia can easily supervene.

Domestic or wild animals

Both domestic pets and rats are likely to be frightened by a building collapse and may attack a rescuer who incautiously presents his or her face through a space.

TYPES OF STRUCTURAL COLLAPSE

The type of collapse depends upon the construction of the building. Framed buildings generally remain standing, even if part of the building is completely destroyed. Debris is usually light. When a total collapse of a framed building does occur, however, the steelwork makes operations extremely difficult.

Unframed buildings collapse in variety of manners, but generally floors tend to survive in large pieces, resulting in the formation of voids upon which the survival of casualties depends.

The 'pancake' collapse

When a supporting wall gives way the upper floor falls onto the lower floor. It seldom falls all the way because heavy furniture, bits of wall, etc., create shallow voids. Often the roof will collapse onto the top of this, leaving the apparent image of an unsurvivable accident (Fig. 12.1). The rescuer who understands the nature of collapse will realise the possibility of survivors, however.

The 'lean-to' collapse

The lean-to collapse occurs when one supporting wall collapses, but the floor is able to support the weight and remain intact, propped against the remaining wall (Fig. 12.2). This type of collapse gives good voids and casualties may even be able to rescue themselves through windows and doors that are unblocked.

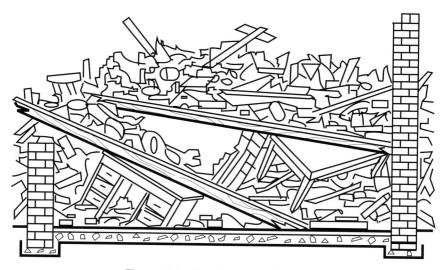

Figure 12.1   Pancake structural collapse.

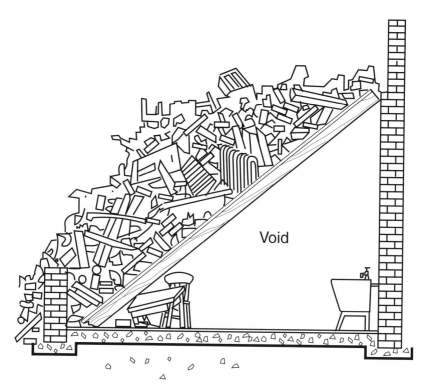

Void

Figure 12.2   Lean-to collapse.

The 'V' collapse

If falling debris from the roof, chimneys or a tower collapses onto the floor, it can break in the middle, creating two voids (Fig. 12.3). In reality, of course, there is often a combination of these types in any multi-floor structural collapse (Fig. 12.4).

RESCUE TECHNIQUES FOR COLLAPSED STRUCTURES

Many of the rescue techniques and procedures for collapsed buildings were devised during the Second World War. They are still as valid today as they were then. Heavy lifting equipment must be used with great caution in a collapsed structure, but some of the modern power saws, acro props and hydraulic rams can be used to great effect in the right circumstances.

The fire service has a clearly defined procedure for dealing with rescue from collapsed buildings. This is divided into five stages.

Stage 1: Reconnaissance and surface casualties

The fire officer reconnoitres the area while the other personnel attend to casualties found in the open. It is important that crews do not indulge in 'debris crawling'. This is the practice of walking on debris. In a collapsed building there is usually a large amount of dust and fine debris that can

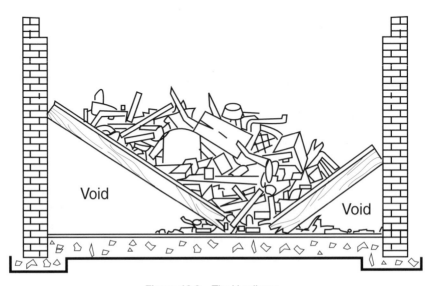

Figure 12.3 The V collapse.

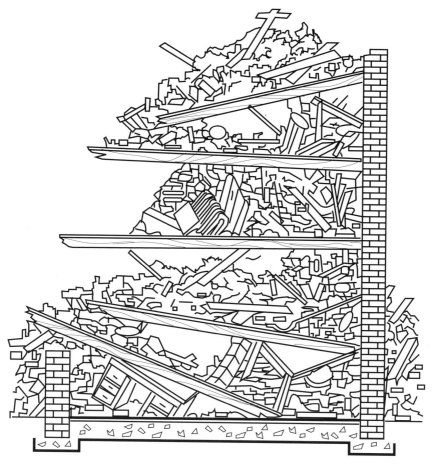

Figure 12.4   A multi-floor collapse.

trickle through the building like sand in an egg timer. Not only can this fill the very voids that are protecting casualties, but the shift of load can destabilise the structure and cause further collapse. This can cause injury and even death to both casualty and rescuer. The loose dust can also pollute the atmosphere in a void and suffocate those trapped.

If casualties, neighbours or bystanders have information, this should be passed to the fire officer. Casualties may want to offer valuable information, and this should be recognised and both rapidly and accurately passed on. On the other hand casualties may not think of providing information unless prompted. The key pieces of information that need to be gained are whether there are any particular hazards involved and where casualties are likely to be found.

Stage 2: Searching slightly damaged buildings

Slightly damaged buildings are those where the roof and floor have not collapsed. These are systematically searched and cleared of casualties. Care in approach and entry to these buildings is important. Floors that are still in position may only be precariously supported and shoring may be required before they can take the load of a rescuer. Buildings should be marked when searched to prevent later teams wasting time searching the same properties again. The letter 'S' near the entrance indicates the building has been searched. This may be further endorsed by adding a '/F' to indicate searched by the fire service, '/P' by police, etc. Where searchers find dangerous conditions, the letter 'D' can also be used after the standard marking. A piece of barricade tape across the entrance will further endorse this. This stage of the rescue should be speedy, but it is imperative that safety precautions are not ignored or serious injury may result.

Rescuers should always work in groups of at least two. Look up before entering for loose slates, damaged chimney stacks or dangerous roofing. Look down to check that the floor is sound underfoot. Do not force doors. It may be that they are merely locked, but the door may be wedged in position because it is bearing a load. If the door is forcibly opened then there may be a further collapse. The best course of action is to find the appropriate window and enter through that. In climbing through the window it is essential to check carefully whether the floor is sound before putting any weight on it. Be very careful climbing through a window that has been damaged by blast. Small fragments of glass can be driven into the woodwork and cause multiple lacerations. Keep close to the walls to minimise the risk of the floor collapsing. Rescuers must remain alert to the signs of further collapse.

Signs of collapse

If faced with entering a collapsed structure to reach a casualty, it is important to realise that incautious movements could trigger further collapse. At all times an awareness needs to be kept of signs that the structure may continue to collapse (see Fig. 12.5). These include:

- sounds of creaking, cracking, crumbling or falling building materials;
- cracked/deformed supporting structures;
- cracked blockwork or render;
- tight doors in frames, particularly if they become so while you are in the building;
- flooding or heavy rain (this can predispose to collapse);
- cratering of the substrate;
- broken glazing, particularly the glass that spontaneously cracks while you are in the building;

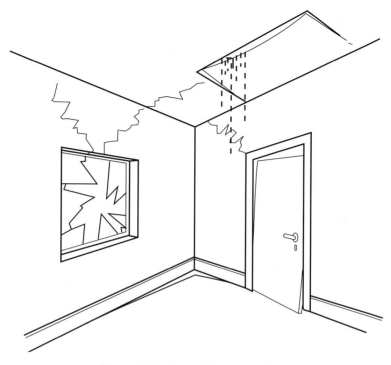

Figure 12.5   Signs of structural collapse.

- sightings out of true;
- loose material, particularly if it starts to fall on you while you are in the building.

Safer places in case of structural collapse

In the event of sudden signs of structural failure the fire service safety officer will give the evacuation signal of short blasts on a whistle. Ideally the building should be vacated immediately, but if bricks and masonry are actually on the move there are several places where you are more likely to survive than others. Doorways are good locations because the structural beam forming the lintel is likely to remain intact. Corners of buildings often withstand collapse, as can columns and archways. Chimney breasts should protect but there is the danger of the chimney collapsing. Staircases are usually good refuges to retreat under.

Stage 3: Searching likely survival points

The piece-by-piece search of a collapsed building can take far longer than an injured and trapped casualty can be expected to survive. The rescuer must enquire as to the likely location of occupants at the time of the collapse. Plans should be consulted if available, and neighbours asked as to occupants' habits. The aim is to search viable and probable locations.

A 'calling and listening period' is appropriate at this stage. All avoidable sound is ceased and the rescue team position themselves around the fringe of the collapsed structure near the position the casualty may be located. They lie on debris and try to get their ears as close as possible to openings that go into the debris. Each person calls out in turn, 'Rescue party – can you hear me?'. All listen intently for sound, and anyone hearing a response indicates with an arm the direction from which the sound appeared to come. It should, however, be remembered that knocking on pipe-work will transmit the sound along a considerable length, and rescue attempts may not be accurately located by this procedure. The fire service have sophisticated acoustic listening devices and thermal imaging equipment that can be deployed rapidly.

Stage 4: Selected debris removal

Framed houses do not usually collapse in their entirety, and thus Stage 4 is usually found in unframed structures. If voice contact is established with the casualty it is important that the first questions are directed to gaining information that will help the formation of a sound extrication plan. How is the person trapped, what hazards are present, are there any openings in the walls in his or her vicinity? This last question may dictate the whole extrication route. Ideally a lane cleared through the debris will be in a straight line to allow easier stretcher handling. If the rescuers come up against a blank wall, however, the rescue is significantly delayed and made more arduous. Once contact has been established it should be maintained at all costs because not only does it keep up morale, but it allows rescuers to check they are heading in the right direction, and the victim can also give warning of any further displacement.

The management of collapsed structures requires a multi-disciplinary approach. Building inspectors and structural engineers may need to be consulted as to the technique of making a building safe. The county council works department may need to be contacted by the police to provide emergency shoring up. Mines rescue and cave rescue teams are experienced in tunnelling and shoring of excavations, and should be considered early.

Entering collapsed structures

Before personnel enter a collapsed structure to treat a casualty prior to and during extrication, certain preparations need to be taken. The route to the casualty will normally have been identified and secured by the fire service, cave rescue or mines rescue, or by a combination of personnel from these

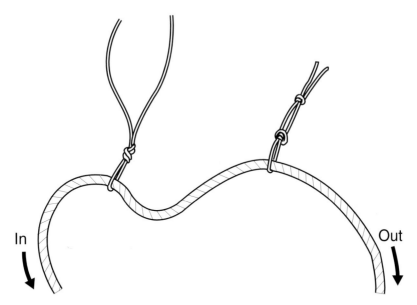

Figure 12.6 A fire service guide line.

teams. A guide line will probably have been laid from the entrance to the casualty. At regular intervals along the line there are two tags that can be easily felt. One tag has two knots, while the other is longer without knots (Fig. 12.6). The line is laid in such a way that it is always possible to tell which direction you are going in, even in total darkness – you can get out by ensuring you are travelling tag to knots. The atmosphere will have been tested and found to be safe, but attention must always be given to the risk of sudden releases of toxic gases or the air become foul due to poor ventilation.

All equipment that enters the environment must be 'intrinsically safe'. This means that there is no possibility of a spark causing an explosion in an inflammable atmosphere. Ideally every rescuer should carry two means of lighting. If one is a helmet lamp, this is ideal. A minimum of equipment should be taken into the environment as space may be severely restricted. It is easier to use several small kit containers rather than one large one. Conversely the stretcher that is used might be better taken into the building fully assembled, as it is certainly going to have to come back out in that condition. Difficulties are best encountered before the casualty is secured to it. Rescue stretchers are not used daily by ambulance and immediate care personnel and therefore familiarisation with the kit before entering is advised.

Attention needs to be paid to the type of clothing required. Exertion in a confined space usually generates such heat that a minimum amount of insulation should be worn. However, if the area has been flooded and a significant amount of time will be spent wet, hypothermia can be the alternative. Wet or even membrane dry suits may be more appropriate.

All personnel should be logged into and out of the structure, working in pairs, and must keep to the guide line, on no account deviating from it. When in the building continually check the integrity of the ground ahead of you before putting your weight on it. Sweep your hand before you with the palm towards you to check there are no dangers in front. By keeping the palm inturned the hand will be thrown free of contact with an electrical current rather than clamp onto it. When the floor slopes away, or appears to drop off, progress should be made feet first, keeping your weight on the solid structure until your feet locate solid ground. If you come across restrictions it is usually wise to progress arms extended, head first, making progress by wriggling and using feet, having previously checked what you will be pushing against. Try to avoid using your arms to pull yourself through as you could displace structures, causing collapse. If you become stuck it is important not to panic. Stop, control your breathing, think about what may have happened and then act appropriately. Panic will cause uncontrolled movements that may cause further collapse.

As you proceed you should relay sufficient information back to your external control for them to construct a map of the interior of the building. This not only provides the ability to set up staging points for equipment, but also allows progress to be related to external structure, thus making warnings of impending collapse more accurate. If you were to become trapped your location would be known. If it is possible to make one member of the team a safety officer this should be done, as it is very easy not to notice signs of further collapse when involved in casualty care.

Stage 5: General debris removal

If there are still casualties to be accounted for after the completion of Stage 4, then the debris is stripped systematically from the site. This is a time-consuming task that has to be started from the perimeter of the collapse. The probability of finding live casualties is low but an ambulance presence will probably be retained at site because of the risks to emergency personnel.

TRENCH COLLAPSE

If called to the scene of a collapsed trench or embankment great care must be taken to ensure that you will not cause further collapse, or further collapse will not entrap you. Soil is heavy, a cubic metre weighing around a ton. Casualties who have the potential of survival either need to be released within minutes to prevent asphyxiation or they will probably be in good enough condition to cope with a protracted extrication. Building regulations and safe working practice are clearly defined for trench construction but regulations may be ignored, mistakes made or the trench may have been constructed by children or do-it-yourself adults. The majority of trench accidents occur in trenches less than 6 feet (2 metres) deep, possibly because the apparent shallowness of the trench leads to complacency. If the accident is due to unforeseen circumstances and the trench has been constructed to the required standard, then part of the structure will probably be intact, giving the rescuers a head start. Often, however, the entire project has been dogged by poor materials, workmanship and judgement and the rescue services are faced with a huge unstable hole in the ground.

The first action of the emergency services must be to move everybody away from the edge of the trench and to turn off any machinery that may cause vibration. If bystanders can see into the trench they are standing too close! It can be very difficult to control a casualty's work mates if they are working frantically when you arrive but, as already said, the casualty will have already expired or will survive a little longer. There may be howls of protest at the turning off of machinery 'that could be useful in the rescue', but vibration sources even 10 or 20 metres away can cause further collapse. However, if the site is well disciplined and the supervisor is obviously competent, then you may decide to let work continue. Always approach a trench at its narrow end, and not from the side. You need to find out the probable location and condition of the victim. Often the casualty will have been pipe laying and may be expected to be found at the point where the new pipes laid beside the trench come to an end. Is the casualty's airway secure? Has any contact been established?

It is necessary to establish what caused the collapse and whether there is any risk of further collapse. Cracks running parallel to the edge of the trench are serious signs. The collapse may have been due to inadequate shoring, the wrong angle of excavation for the type of soil, the soil structure changing as a result of heavy rain, vibration from machinery, or excessive loading of the edge of the trench due to spoil piles (which can increase in weight with rainfall), or crowding of the edge with on-lookers. You need to know what risks there are within the trench. Water, sewage or gas pipes may have been fractured in the collapse and need to be isolated. Power cables carrying anything from 415 to 33 000 volts may have been damaged. It is possible that the atmosphere at the bottom of a trench may be non-respirable. If any of these hazards exist, or if the shoring appears less than competently done, entry to the trench should not be considered.

A casualty's colleagues can be set to work protecting the edges of the trench with large plywood sheets to spread the load of the rescuers. If a spoil pile gets in the way it will need moving back from the edge, a laborious task, yet one that may be vital as the rescue progresses.

Recently legal precedent has been established that deems the emergency services to be acting within their remit of 'to save life' by suspending rescue operations if the rescuers are in serious danger.

KEY POINT

- A successful rescue relies on careful planning and training before entering the structure.

Self-test questions for Chapter 12

1. State two reasons why the oxygen level in a confined space might be reduced and give two ways in which the rescuers may overcome this problem.

2. What are the constituents of sewer gas?

3. Give four domestic hazards that a rescuer in a collapsed building may face.

4. What three things may occur while you are within a building that would lead you to expect imminent collapse?

5. What is the particular requirement of electrical equipment used in a confined space?

6. What are the early symptoms of carbon monoxide poisoning?

7. What is 'debris crawling' and what are the dangers of doing it?

8. Where might casualties be expected to be found alive in a collapsed building?

9. Which way is out when using a fire service guide line?

10. While crawling through a collapsed building your foot becomes entangled. What should you do?

Answers on p. 212.

Casualty evacuation in difficult terrain

Difficult terrain covers a multitude of options. The use of specialist teams should be considered. In most counties these consist of:

- police air support unit
- county air ambulance
- RAF Search & Rescue helicopters
- fire service rope rescue team
- mountain rescue team
- cliff rescue team
- the coastguard
- RNLI (Royal National Lifeboat Institution)
- cave rescue team
- mines rescue team.

It is important to understand the strengths and weaknesses of each team to make the best use of the services these groups offer.

HELICOPTER RESCUE TEAMS

Police air support unit

Under their responsibility to save life the police of many counties will, if requested by the ambulance service, allow their helicopter to be used for the transport of the injured. Available ostensibly 24 hours a day, in fact there is usually down time due to servicing, shift problems and weather. The police may well need the helicopter in their criminal detection role and so this service cannot be relied upon.

Most police helicopters can carry one casualty only, in circumstances that make intervention in an emergency almost impossible. The receiving hospital should have approved helicopter landing facilities close to the A&E department. Flying time to the hospital from anywhere in the county is unlikely to be in excess of 20 minutes. There is little available payload so the heavier the patient, the lighter the attendant and equipment must be. There is usually no winch facility but, by keeping the rotors going, it is possible to accept casualties from very soft terrain. There is a considerable hazard when undertaking this type of recovery. The pilot has the right to abort any mission for safety reasons. Standard helicopter landing requirements (see Box 13.1) apply.

County air ambulances

In an increasing number of counties journey time to the incident and the hospital can be substantially reduced by the use of an air ambulance. These helicopters are usually designed to allow good access to the casualty in case of an in-flight emergency. They have similar problems as the police helicopters with regard to night landing, weather and servicing. They also usually only carry one casualty, though most can theoretically carry two. They will be mobilised as the primary response in circumstances of difficult patient access such as moorland or fell. They may be mobilised at the request of a road ambulance crew if the casualty is considered time critical, there is poor road access to the most appropriate receiving unit, or there is a high probability of a spinal injury. Air ambulances are unsuitable for infectious cases, psychiatric cases and obstetric cases when birth is imminent.

The helicopter will usually land and 'power down' over a couple of minutes and ensure the rotors have stopped before allowing personnel to

---

Box 13.1   Landing site preparation

The site should be clear of tall obstacles.

The actual landing spot should be firm and at least 15 metres in diameter.

The maximum slope should be no more than 12°.

An area of 100 metres should be cleared around the landing site.

Indicate the wind direction if possible.

Keep the area clear of people, loose material and animals.

approach. The process of stopping and then re-starting the rotors takes around 4 minutes. If seconds are vital, the pilot may sanction a 'hot load', in which the rotors are kept going. It is essential that the precise instructions of the crew are followed to avoid accidents.

RAF and coastguard search and rescue helicopters

These helicopters are primarily mobilised from RAF bases with a flight time of approximately 35–40 minutes. They have a winching facility and can take several casualties. They can carry a substantial payload. Always follow the directions of the crew.

RAF helicopters have night vision capability. Never shine a torch directly at a helicopter at night. It is unlikely you would actually cause a crash, but you could temporarily blind the pilots and they may well abort the rescue because of the danger you cause.

Helicopters can build up a significant static charge and a winchline should be allowed to ground itself before being touched. If you have to be winched using a strop, then it should be placed under both arms, adjusted, and then the arms kept to the sides during winching. The helicopter crew will bring you into the aircraft when you reach the top of the hoist. Once removed from the hoist go to the seat indicated and strap in. Handles and levers marked in black and yellow stripes are emergency release mechanisms and must never be used as hand holds.

General principles of helicopter safety (Fig. 13.1)

Rotors

Normal practice is to embark/disembark with the rotor blades stationary and the line of approach should always be within the 'safe area'. Do not approach the helicopter until you are given a 'thumbs-up' sign from the pilot. You will be accompanied throughout this procedure by a crew member.

Should circumstances dictate, passengers may embark/disembark with the rotor blades turning, but only with the pilot's permission and strictly according to instructions. You should remain within the 'safe area' and await a 'thumbs-up' signal. Never approach or leave from the uphill side. Carry tools or equipment below the waist and make sure chinstraps are secure on helmets.

Do not slam the doors on helicopters; close them gently and do not let them swing in the wind.

Seat belts

Seat belts should be fastened at all times, ensuring they are **tightly** secured prior to take off. Do not unfasten until rotor blades have stopped.

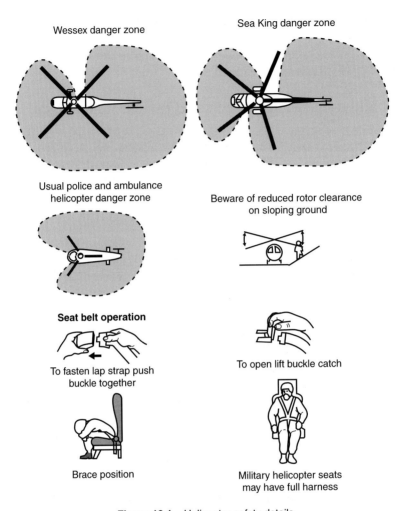

Figure 13.1 Helicopter safety details.

Doors

Once the doors have been closed and secured, do not attempt to open them until the helicopter has landed, and then only with the pilot's permission. The door operation varies from aircraft to aircraft. If not familiar with the system, allow a member of the crew to open the door for you. Some doors can actually be jettisoned if you pull the wrong bit! The crew will not be amused by this action.

Loose articles

Ensure you are not in possession of loose articles that could fall from pockets. If anything is dropped you should **inform a crew member immediately**.

Comfort while travelling in a helicopter

Fitness to fly

If you are suffering from a cold, an ear or sinus infection or are an epileptic taking medication, you should not fly.

Ventilation/heating

In civilian helicopters it may be possible for the pilot to adjust the ventilation for your, or the patient's, comfort, but you will need to ask. Fresh air vents positioned above your head can be used. Additionally, the temperature of the cabin can be controlled if you advise the pilot.

Air sickness

You should inform the pilot or other crew member if you feel unwell. Should you require them, discomfort bags are generally available. Some people find the flicker effect generated by the rotors very disturbing as it induces a form of vertigo.

Helicopter in-flight emergencies

Helicopters are not as safe as passenger aircraft. Emergencies, however, are reasonably rare. In the unlikely event of an emergency the pilot will do his or her best to keep you informed. However, the pilot will not want you to engage in conversation. Your seat belt may be needed so you should not loosen seat belts or open doors until the helicopter is stationary on the ground. You should observe the position of emergency exits and handles as you may need to operate them yourself. Be prepared to adopt the brace position. Try not to hold your breath.

If you are involved in over-water flights you will be required to wear a life jacket. If an emergency occurs and a landing in water is made, **do not inflate the jacket** inside the aircraft.

FIRE AND RESCUE SERVICE

The fire and rescue service can provide basic equipment to assist access to difficult locations. The principal resource is the ladders they carry. It is not uncommon for emergency personnel other than firefighters to be required to climb ladders.

Using ladders safely

Firefighter terminology of ladders appears to be related to rope ladders, and therefore probably originates from the navy. The sides of the ladder are known as strings and the cross pieces are called rounds. The top of a ladder is called the head and the bottom is called the heel. Ladders must always be held in place before they are climbed. They may be tied to a solid and unmoving object or they may be held in place at the bottom by someone for the entire duration that there is somebody on the ladder. This is known as footing the ladder. Before stepping onto a ladder a firefighter will call, 'Foot the ladder!' And the person responsible for the task will reply, 'Ladder footed'. If using fire service ladders you should follow this discipline.

Ladders should be climbed using both hands and both feet (Fig. 13.2). If anything needs to be carried up the ladder it should be put over the shoul-

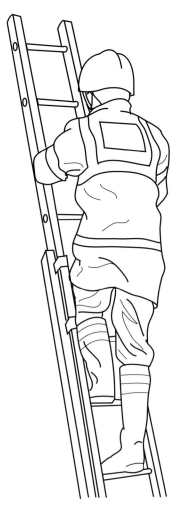

Figure 13.2 The correct way to climb a ladder.

ders, or tied to the waist. Hands and feet are always placed on the rounds. If the climber loses his or her foothold and hands are only gripping the strings, then there is a risk of sliding down the ladder. When climbing ladders the hands and feet should move in unison, i.e. right hand, right foot, left hand, left foot. The arms should be kept reasonably straight with the body away from the ladder. As a general guide, the climber should grasp the round level with the chest, with the palms down and the thumb underneath. When climbing extension ladders there are stages when the rounds of one section overlie the rounds of another. Only grip one round at a time. To try to grip both means that the hand cannot be closed effectively and there is a greater risk of slipping. Always climb so that alternate hands and feet are in contact with the rounds. Look forwards or up; looking down can frequently cause vertigo.

On reaching the head of the ladder, it is usually necessary to dismount to one side or the other. The correct technique will be described for dismounting to the left of the ladder (Fig. 13.3), but dismounting to the right merely requires swapping the roles of the hands and feet. Regaining the ladder is a direct reversal of dismounting.

While gripping a round with the right hand, take the left hand around the left string and grip a round with the palm turned uppermost. This enables the left leg to be placed over the windowsill or balustrade. Before transferring your weight entirely to the left foot, use it to test the integrity of the floor, then transfer the right leg over, release the right hand, and finally the left hand.

ROPE RESCUE

Traditional rope techniques

As the result of recent policy changes regarding entry into confined spaces, particularly sewers and silos, the fire service are abandoning the age-old procedure of a rope with a bowline tied around the rescuer. Simple access systems of full body harness, rope, tripod and hand winch are to be introduced onto incident support units. Modern studies have confirmed that severe respiratory embarrassment occurs when hanging from a bowline and death can occur within an hour. It is therefore not a procedure for vertical lowering. It does, however, retain a use for improvised safety lines on steep slopes, but not cliff faces.

Fire service rope rescue team

Most fire services have a rope rescue team. They have equipment that will allow the evacuation of casualties from all situations that require rope access, e.g. from inaccessible parts of buildings, cranes and gantries. Their

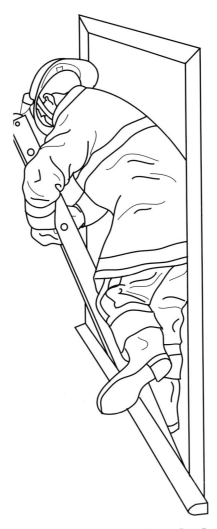

Figure 13.3 How to dismount from the top (head) of a ladder.

response time obviously depends on the location of the incident within the county, but may be 30–40 minutes. Setting up the necessary rope-work may take another 30 minutes.

Mountain rescue teams

Mountain rescue teams carry extensive ropes and stretcher equipment suitable for the 'carry-off' of casualties from moorland, fell and crag, or from situations where the rope rescue team may also be deployed. The advantage of the mountain rescue team is the number of team members who are available, as a difficult and prolonged carry-off may need up to 30 team members. The disadvantage, however, is the relatively slow response to a call-out. Significant numbers are likely to be achieved only after an hour has elapsed.

Rescue ropes

Ambulances in some counties have recently been equipped with 100-foot (~30 metres) ropes to act as a safety line if necessary. The ropes are intended to help crew descend, ascend and traverse steep slopes safely, and also as a safety line in the case of water rescue.

It is extremely important that all personnel understand a few basic concepts about rope handling and management. The overall goal is to maximise the life of the rope as well as the life of the person dangling from the end of it. With this in mind, everyone should take pains to avoid jumping, walking or sitting on a rope. Dragging a rope on the ground allows small dirt particles to become embedded in the sheath, work their way into the core, and slowly cut fibres. Do not leave rope under tension for any extended period unless absolutely necessary. Remove all knots as soon as possible and try to avoid overloading a knot at all costs. A wet rope is demonstrably weaker and harder to handle than a dry one.

Nylon rope is very resistant to petrol, grease and oil but is very rapidly damaged by battery acid, bleach and other electrolytes. This damage can occur within 15 minutes of exposure and substantially weakens the rope with very little indication but for a stiffening of the sheath. Any rope that has been exposed to acids should be condemned. Dirty ropes should be washed in accordance with the manufacturer's guidance but should never be dried in front of a fire, as high temperatures also damage rope. Heat can be generated by friction of nylon moving across nylon. Kinking of rope should be avoided if possible, because if stressed while kinked, severe damage can result. Any rope subjected to damage should be reported as damaged and removed from service. To use a rope to tow a vehicle and then return it to service may cause the death of a colleague many months later.

A rescue rope is checked by careful inspection of the sheath while the rope is uncoiled. Be aware of how the rope feels to the fingers; if enough central strands rupture a localised reduction in diameter can be detected. Check any suspect areas under body weight tension. It must be realised that without the use of a mountaineering harness the rope is inappropriate for lowering personnel. It must also be realised that a safety rope does not protect an individual from the severe and potentially life-threatening physiological changes that occur when a body at 37°C enters water at least 25°C lower. Immersion in cold water can cause ventricular tachycardia or fibrillation. These are not cardiac rhythms that are compatible with the survival of a rescuer. A rope does not protect a life, merely recovers a body.

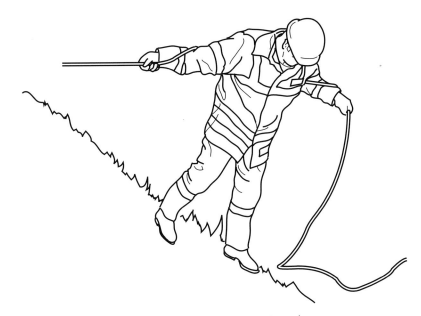

Figure 13.4   Using a rope on a steep slope.

Having said this, a rope is also only as secure as the point to which it is attached. Since every action has an equal and opposite reaction, if one ambulance worker is thrown away from a static person of similar mass, then both will be moved. **Always** secure the end of the rope to something that **will not** move. The rope **may** be used for a hand hold on a steep slope where the majority of the load can be carried on the ground surface. The rope should be secured at the top of the slope and is used most effectively when the rope is passed over the shoulders, given a half turn around both arms, and controlled through both gloved hands (Fig. 13.4). Looking straight down the slope and, keeping the legs straight, a brisk walk down hill is undertaken. To stop the downhill arm is brought across the chest and the grip secured.

On steeper slopes the rope must be tied to the ambulance worker. A bowline is the most appropriate knot. Rope is elastic and does stretch under load up to 30%. Ropes should be kept with the minimum of slack if a fall may have to be arrested.

Useful knots

To tie a bowline it is easiest to remember the method that taught many generations of boy scouts. Wrap the rope around your waist. Make a loop in the rope length that represents a rabbit hole with a tree trunk behind it. The end of the rope is the rabbit. It pops out of the hole, sees you, runs behind the tree, and then decides to run back down the hole again (Fig. 13.5).

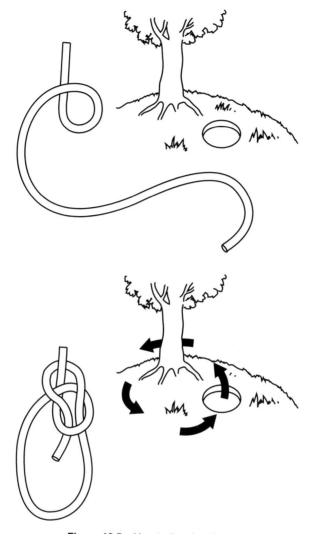

Figure 13.5   How to tie a bowline.

A second valuable knot is the figure of eight (Fig. 13.6). This allows a length of rope to be secured to an anchor point even if both ends are unavailable.

Finally, a third useful knot is also shown (Fig. 13.7). This allows one person to control the lowering of another with ease. Tension applied to the lower end in the diagram will prevent movement of the upper rope. A release of tension allows the rope to feed out.

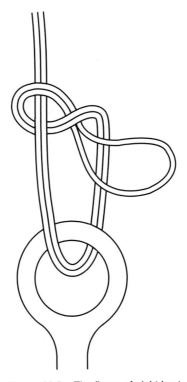

Figure 13.6 The figure of eight knot.

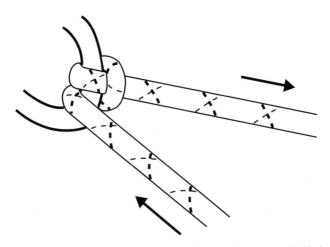

Figure 13.7 Italian or Munter hitch – a useful knot for a controlled belay.

When to rope-up

There are no hard and fast rules about when to rope-up. This is a decision that is influenced by a number of interrelated factors:

1. Exposure – would a slip result in serious injury?
2. Difficulty – is the terrain difficult to a degree that makes a slip a possibility?
3. Ability – how do individual rescuers react to exposure and how do they perform on rock?
4. Security – can the situation be properly safeguarded by the use of the rope?
5. The time factor – speed is often a safety factor in itself. Is the saving of time more important under the circumstances than the additional security that can be provided by roping-up?
6. Margin of safety – even in an emergency situation, rescuers must be operating within their experience and capabilities.

If, having weighed these factors, you decide to rope-up, you must see to it that the rope is used as effectively and efficiently as possible.

Sound belaying is the only key to safe practice in this area. This depends on the selection of a safe and suitable anchor for the rope and on a thorough appreciation both in theory and practice of the technique of belaying.

Anchors

The selection of a really solid anchor is the first essential in setting up a belay system. It cannot be considered in isolation, although it is likely to be the determining factor in locating the belay. Ideally the anchor should take a pull from any direction, e.g. an ambulance towing point or a tree. Sometimes only one anchor and belay position is possible; at others you may have a limited choice. Choose the best position from which you can safeguard the person climbing (Fig. 13.8).

You should be able to follow the climber's progress on the pitch so that you can offer advice and encouragement. The rope needs to be kept clear of loose debris so that it does not get dislodged and fall on the climber. The rope should not run over any sharp edges or it will become frayed and dangerous.

You should have sufficient room to adopt a good sitting position, with a firm brace for the feet. The position of the belayer should, if possible, be in the same vertical plane as the climber and the anchor. This is because if the climber falls the rope will tend to straighten between the climber and the anchor, and if they are not in a straight line, the belayer will be pulled sideways.

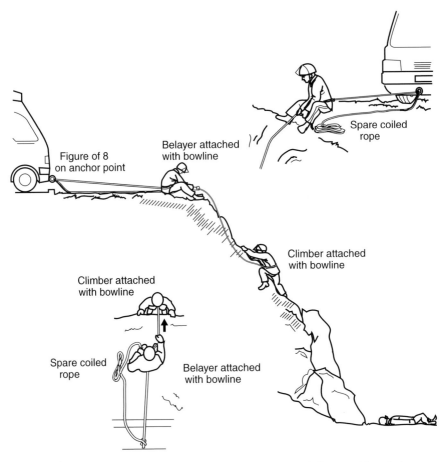

Belayer attached with bowline

Figure of 8 on anchor point

Spare coiled rope

Climber attached with bowline

Climber attached with bowline

Spare coiled rope

Belayer attached with bowline

Figure 13.8   Three views showing the use of an anchor, a belayer and the climber.

Attachment of the belayer to the anchor

Both the climber and the belayer attach themselves to opposite ends of the rope by a bowline. The belayer then measures the distance to the anchor point, and ties the rope to the anchor point with a figure of eight so that the rope is taut when the belay position is adopted. The belayer cannot then be pulled onto the climbing face. The belayer should wear protective gloves. With the rest of the climbing rope at one side the belayer passes the rope over his or her head and down to the hips. The inactive rope is twisted once around the forearm before being held firmly in the braking hand.

As the climber descends the active rope should be kept under just the right degree of tension so that at no time is there any slack rope between the belayer and the rescuer. In the event of a slip the rope is held tightly in the braking hand, which is moved across the front of the body so as to provide maximum friction between rope and hips. Even a short fall can impose a tremendous load on the belayer that can test his or her strength and skill.

WATER AND ICE RESCUE

Remember the principle of water rescue is to **Reach, Throw, Wade, Row,** and only finally consider **Swim & Tow**. In other words, if you can reach out to someone while you are secure on the bank, even if this means using a stretcher pole or similar device, then you should do so. If you cannot reach this way, then you should consider throwing a life buoy or a throwing rope. If you can wade out to the person without losing your footing, this is the next option, but be wary of unseen drop-offs or underwater dangers. If you can use a boat do so, but a small dinghy can capsize if a panicking individual tries to clamber aboard incorrectly. Only if all other options are exhausted should you consider swimming out to the victim and trying to tow him or her back. You need to be a very strong swimmer who is well trained in life saving techniques. If ropes are used incorrectly they can be the cause of the rescuer's death. If faced with a water rescue you should first assess the scene. Is the water still, fast-flowing or tidal? What is the bottom composition? Where is the exit route? It needs experience to read water, but there are a few basic principles. You may well decide that without specialist training and equipment you would be unwise to attempt a rescue.

Fast-flowing water

The pattern of water velocity varies along the route of a water course; some of the features of fast-flowing water are illustrated in Figure 13.9. In general, water in a channel flows faster in the centre and on the surface than along the shores and bottom. Water flows faster on the outside of a turn, resulting in a locally deeper channel and undercut banks, whereas the inside of a bend has slower-moving shallower water by comparison. At the beginning of rapids a number of smooth waves form as water channels itself to flow through areas free of obstruction. The *tongues* indicate the safest route for the paddler to enter the area as water is deep and free of obstructions. Fixed *standing waves* indicate the water has been diverted vertically by an underwater obstruction, but probably the most dangerous areas are *hydraulics*, which are formed by water crashing over an underwater obstruction in such a way that it curls upwards and back on itself. The most serious hydraulics occur at dams, waterfalls and weirs. Hydraulics can easily trap a body, and are often too dangerous to search. They are easily identified by the way floating debris circles in one spot instead of moving rapidly downstream.

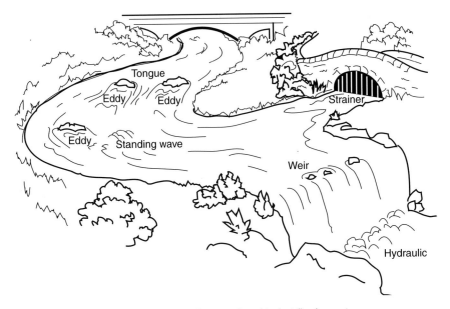

Figure 13.9 Various features found in fast-flowing water.

At any place along a water course a *strainer* may occur. This is anything that combs the water passing through it, but blocks the passage of an object in the current and pins it to the strainer by the pressure of the water. *Eddies* are pockets of calm water, located on the downstream side of obstructions. A vacuum is created by fast-moving water flowing around the obstacle, creating a haven of calm water in the midst of the flow.

As you enter the water by wading out more and more of your body weight is supported by the water. Generally by the time you are knee deep there is not enough downward force on the bottom from your weight to prevent you being swept away by anything greater than a gentle current. Because of this rescuers should not enter the water further than up to their knees unless properly equipped with a wetsuit, a belay and a personal flotation device (PFD).

Rescue in the 'white water' environment in the UK is time critical. If the water is near freezing then a casualty will have less than 5 minutes useful work before hypothermia sets in and less than 15 minutes to unconsciousness. In the summer and autumn this may be up to 7.5 minutes and 30 minutes, respectively. Immersing a hot person in cold water can cause immediate cardiac arrest.

If a search is required then it is most prudent for the first responder to establish a confinement boundary by multiplying the time that has elapsed by the river's velocity and dispatching look-outs to an appropriate stretch of slower water downstream. A 'hasty search' is conducted as a quick survey for someone in immediate danger, hanging to a rock or branch. Look in eddies and strainers for equipment or clothing as clues. Detailed searches in white water are effectively for the recovery of bodies and not the remit of this book.

Tidal water

In the British Isles there are two periods of high water and two of low water in each lunar day (about 24 hours and 50 minutes), although tides vary locally. The difference in the height of the water between successive high and low waters is called the range of the tide. In the British Isles the range of the tide can vary from as little as 1–2 metres to as much as 10 metres in some places. The time between successive high waters is about half a lunar day (i.e. about 12 hours 24 minutes).

The greatest range of tide is found at or near the full moon. These are called spring tides and occur about every 15 days throughout the year. About midway between spring tides the sun and moon are at right angles to the earth and the smallest range of tides is found at this time. These are called neap tides. Greater than average spring tides will be found near the equinoxes (March and September), and higher tides will occur in areas where there is a strong on-shore prevailing wind.

The tide rises or falls at a given site according to the rule of twelfths, as outlined in Box 13.2. This information, as well as a knowledge of high tide, is of importance when working anywhere below the high water mark. It should also be remembered that all operations that take place below the high water mark are under the jurisdiction of the coastguard.

As the tide rises or falls large masses of water have to move, and this gives rise to tide streams. In areas where this water has to pass through a narrow channel the currents can be very strong indeed, and in estuaries that are relatively flat and narrow markedly from mouth to tidal limit a moving wall of water (a bore) can be created. Large flat bays do not create a bore, but the sea can cross the sands faster than a man can run. Where the tidal currents of two masses of water meet and fight against each other,

---

Box 13.2 The rule of twelfths

The tide will rise or fall, as appropriate, as follows:
- 1/12th of the range in the first sixth of its duration
- 2/12ths of the range in the second sixth of its duration
- 3/12ths of the range in the third sixth of its duration
- 3/12ths of the range in the fourth sixth of its duration
- 2/12ths of the range in the fifth sixth of its duration
- 1/12th of the range in the final sixth of its duration

such as at a prominent headland, a tidal rip is formed. Small boats can have great difficulty in these waters and swimmers are in great danger.

In narrow channels with sand or mud banks to either side strong shore-ward currents may be created as the tide rises. On a beach with an off-shore sand bank water driven over the bar by wave action has to return by any opening as the wave ebbs. This gives rise to strong off-shore currents in localised areas. These rip currents will sweep the unwary out to sea.

When in the sea there is usually the problem of getting out. On a beach the retreating wave creates a strong undertow that not only pulls a swimmer back, but also destabilises the sand or shale on which the swimmer stands. When climbing out on rock waves tend to throw the swimmer first against the rock and then suddenly retreat, depositing all the body weight onto sharp, slippery and treacherous hand holds. All too frequently rescuers are battered by waves against rocks until they weaken or are knocked uncon-scious. Even putting all the dangers inherent with the swimming rescue techniques aside, the environmental difficulties of the sea must make any attempt of saving life at sea by an unequipped amateur an almost certain fatal failure.

Black water

Black water refers to any water with very limited or zero visibility due to the turbidity of the water. The dangers are in two forms. First, the particu-late matter that reduces the visibility may be harmful to health, either as a biological agent, as in raw sewage for example, or less likely, it may be a chemical toxin. The possibility of contracting Weil's disease from a water course infested by rats must not be forgotten, and after any rescue in these conditions the advice of the environmental health department should be taken.

The greater danger to the rescuer lies in what may be concealed by the water. Black water often hides a multitude of hazards in the form of steel cable, pipes, supermarket trolleys, broken glass, wrecked vehicles, etc., all of which may injure or ensnare the rescuer. Since most of these items are thrown in from the side, and often into slow-moving water, they may rest in an unstable position until kicked by the swimmer, who then becomes entangled. If they then settle in a significantly deeper location, the rescuer goes too. There can be no justification in attempting to locate a body under-water in black water by anyone but the police underwater search team.

Ice

Every year people die when they fall through the ice on lakes or rivers. The dramatic stories of full recovery after drowning in icy water spur on the rescuers to unprecedented levels of stupidity. A little thought about the mechanics of ice will reveal the dangers. Ice is always thicker at the edge of the lake, the centre of the lake being the last to freeze. It is the same for rivers, but the problem here is compounded by the fact that as the cold weather continues there is less rainfall running off into the river and so the water level falls, leaving the ice unsupported underneath. In estuaries salt water, which has a lower freezing point, will twice daily circulate below the ice to assist its thaw.

Rubbish and branches that rest on the surface act as score lines along which ice can fracture, and it is the integrity of an intact sheet of ice that allows it to support weight at all. As an increasing load is applied the ice initially behaves like a beam of wood. There is a degree of bending and the load is spread throughout the ice. If one edge is unsupported then the load is no longer spread evenly, but is applied more like a lever. As soon as the load exceeds a critical limit, the ice will no longer bend but will crack.

There are five ways of dealing with the problem of thin ice. The first possibility, which relies on the casualty still clinging to the edge of the ice, is to throw a rope to the casualty and hope the casualty is still able to get his or her arms into a bowline pre-tied into it. The technique for rope throwing is described in Box 13.3. Some fire services have connectors that allow fire hose to be inflated with compressed air to become fairly rigid and buoyant.

Failing this, a structure such as a ladder is placed from edge to edge and supported on land, and the rescue effected from the safety of the ladder. If this technique is used the ladder must be secured at both ends and a short safety line should be used to attach the rescuer to the ladder. The largest ladder routinely available to the fire service is 13.5 metres. Turntable ladders and aerial platforms are longer, but there may well be problems of access close to the water owing to soft ground, problems of stability due to ground sloping towards the water, and the problem of stability if the fully extended ladder is taken beyond its safe working perimeter.

Alternatively a platform that will float may be used, ideally an inflatable dinghy (a proper size, not a beach toy). There is still the risk that breaking ice sheets may tip the dinghy, so crew need to be protected with dry suits and personal flotation devices. A suitable dinghy is usually available to the fire service.

Box 13.3 Technique for throwing a rope

Make sure the rope is neatly coiled. Split the coil into two and take one half in your left hand and the other in your right. Gain some momentum with a swinging motion of your right arm and then let go the right-hand coil with a forward fling. As it flakes out ahead, let the left-hand coil follow. Extra momentum can be gained by tying the two head blocks from a head immobiliser to the end of the rope.

The fourth, and least desirable, technique is to spread the weight of the rescuer over as much ice as possible. A 9-year-old child weighs approximately 50 kg and will have, when standing, applied their whole load over 400 cm^2. This is a load of 125 g/cm^2. An average adult weighs 70 kg, and spreading this weight evenly over the entire surface of a long board would only be exerting a load of 50 g/cm^2. Before this apparently easy solution is adopted, however, the drawbacks must be considered. The integrity of the ice has been damaged by the casualty; the weight of the long board has not been considered; and, more importantly, the end loading in the struggle to get the casualty onto the board would almost certainly exceed the load limit of the ice at the edge of the break.

The final possibility depends on location, but relies on a helicopter being able to either winch or hover with a observer on the skid to grab the casualty. Even though this may be the only time-viable life-saving alternative, it must be at the discretion of the crew.

SNOW SAFETY

Every winter lives are lost in mountainous areas where snow falls. Avalanche and blizzard are recognised as threats to safety. Management of rescues in country terrain during heavy snow is a specialist subject and the reader is referred to the various texts on mountain rescue (for example Langmuir 1995). Snow in urban areas can also be a source of risk. Leaving aside the risk that driving in snow causes, the principal problem of snow is that it covers a multitude of hazards in the same way that a foam blanket does (Fig. 13.10). What appears to be a gentle slope may be a steep drop softened by wind-blown snow. Sharp objects and unstable surfaces may all be hidden. What appears to be the edge of a drop may be an overhang that can give way. Snow can rest easily on surfaces that act as a slide when the unwary walk on them. As the person starts to slide he or she can start a mini-avalanche. Lives have been lost where walkers have suddenly lost their footing, slid over a ledge, been injured on the ground below, and covered by the snow they have disturbed.

Hypothermia

Loss of body heat is well recognised as a problem for the casualty who is lying immobile and shocked in a cold environment. It is less well recognised as a complication of warm but windy weather, and only rarely does the rescuer realise the problem of hypothermia can affect them as well.

The human being endeavours to maintain a constant body temperature. In hot climates the body attempts to lose heat by the evaporation of sweat. In cold climates the body tries to generate heat by shivering or by allowing the outside of the body to cool, preserving a core of normal body tem-

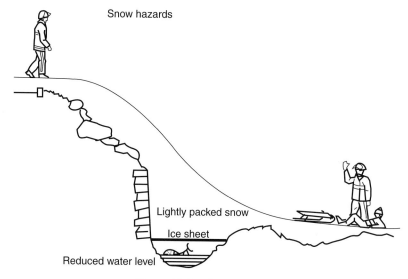

Figure 13.10   Snow hazards.

perature. Hypothermia occurs when the core temperature cannot be maintained and the body's metabolism begins to slow.

It is the combination of exhaustion, cold, and mental stress that is particularly dangerous. Two major factors affect the body's cooling: windchill and wet cold.

Windchill

Just as the blushing Victorian debutante cools herself with a fan, so wind cools the body. This is most marked at low wind speeds, as everyone who welcomes a gentle breeze on a sultry summer day will testify. A good windproof garment is essential to avoiding windchill. Unfortunately ambulance crews and police officers are often given half-length jackets that are windproof and waterproof, but no protection is offered to the legs. The wearing of a helmet is important as it reduces heat loss from the body by nearly 10%. All firefighters will testify to the beneficial effects of their flash-hoods in bad weather. These items of dress can usually be obtained from the fire service by either formal or informal arrangements.

Wet cold

Even the best clothing suffers an enormous loss of its insulating efficiency when it becomes wet, as water is a hundred times better a conductor of heat than air. Evaporation robs the clothing of even more heat. After all, this is the mechanism by which water puts out fires.

Symptoms of hypothermia

Severe hypothermia is unlikely to occur in the team approach to incident management. Mild hypothermia can creep up on the unwary rescuer, however, causing a variety of symptoms that will impede the safe completion of the task. The first sign is usually unexpected and apparently unreasonable behaviour, often with complaints of coldness and tiredness. There may be a degree of lethargy and failure to respond to questions and directions. Unexpected outbursts of ill-directed energy, swearing and lack of insight into the creeping cold can all occur. This is the worst stage that rescuers are likely to encounter themselves. Usually by then the casualty has been evacuated. The vehicle driver may not be fit to drive, and the extent of the exhaustion may not be appreciated. Even if the casualty safely reaches hospital, the pressures on the control staff may be pushing the crew back onto the road before they have recovered. Control officers need to appreciate the potential for hypothermia and be prepared to mobilise senior officers to supervise the physical needs of crews whenever the potential for hypothermia can occur.

SAND AND MUD RESCUE

People have been getting stuck and perishing in quicksand throughout time and, even today, with all the technology we have around us, we still struggle to try to rescue people with very basic implements. In an incident at Morecambe Bay, Lancashire, in August 1997, fire service and the coastguard had to resort to using their bare hands to try to dig the casualty out.

We need to understand what quicksand is, how it works, and how to overcome its effect, so that we can be effective in our efforts. There are basically two different types of ground or earth that are capable of trapping people or animals: quicksand and mud flats. Quicksand consists of liquid and sand particles that are mobile, i.e. capable of moving, but they can also compress around a person or object and hold them. Mud flats are a lot less mobile than quicksand but still can exert a hold on people. With mud flats, usually someone gets stuck and if not rescued will perish because of the cold or the incoming tide. We must be aware that these two types of earth hold people in different ways, and, because of this, different methods of rescue are required.

With mud flats the casualty or victim is held in place by a vacuum effect. Therefore the only way to release them is to break the vacuum by introducing air as close to the casualty as possible. This will release the vacuum and therefore the casualty. This is where the fire service mud or sand lance comes in. This is a long hollow steel spike with side holes to permit the release of compressed air. It is inserted as close to the victim as possible and pressurised from compressed air bottles. However, what happens when the only piece of equipment we have for this type of rescue proves to be inadequate? This is what occurred at Morecambe. If air does not work, then the other alternative is water.

Quicksand differs from mud. In quicksand as the casualty moves, the sand particles are forced apart, allowing water in between them and making them more liquid, so the person sinks even more and makes the situation worse. Quicksand has to be considered as a liquid. People can float on it, but they must adopt a swimming position before they sink too deeply in it to be able to change position from vertical to horizontal.

When victims do not react quickly enough they become trapped. This is because pressure from above compacts the sand lower down, effectively gripping the casualty. This compacted sand must be released somehow. The current method is to insert the sand lance as deep as possible and to inject air. Unfortunately, the sand lance may not be located in the correct position below the casualty. When air is injected around the casualty's legs, the sand particles are forced apart. However, as the air rises to the surface it is replaced by water. This either makes the sand around the casualty's legs more mobile and fluid, allowing the casualty to sink a little more, or the action of the air compresses the sand even more, merely increasing the grip on the casualty.

In more silty or sandy types of sediment the injection of air has potential for release, but the air needs to be retained to give buoyancy. Otherwise it simply rises to the surface and causes further liquefaction. The answer is to increase the water pressure around the person's feet, forcing the particles apart and releasing the compacted and interlocked sediment particles from around the feet and legs. The sand lance has therefore been adapted to use both air and water. When doing this the victim must be prevented from sinking further.

The incident at Morecambe highlighted areas that need to be addressed. The first priority is the safety of the rescuers, and one safety item is an inflatable walkway that can allow rescuers to reach and work with the casualty without risk of them becoming trapped. Another innovation is a method of preventing removed sediment from flowing back around the casualty. This will take the form of a metal box, open at the top and bottom, that will go over the casualty and can be forced down around him or her. This is just like shoring or shuttering, and will give the rescuers more time.

In addition, an item that will relieve rescuers from the fatigue of getting their own feet constantly stuck is a device called a 'Mudbuster'. It fits onto the fireboot and basically lets air enter at the base of the boot, releasing the suction around the boot.

KEY POINTS

- Rescue ropes do not necessarily save life, they merely aid the recovery of a body.
- Use specialist rescue teams when required.

Self-test questions for Chapter 13

1. At what point is it safe to approach a helicopter?

2. Where is the 'no-go' area of a helicopter?

3. How big should a landing area for a helicopter be?

4. What is the length of the ambulance service rescue rope?

5. State four circumstances when roping up would be appropriate.

6. What are the components of an effective roping system for steep slopes?

7. Give four factors that govern the position of the belayer.

8. What is the sequence of options in water rescue?

9. What devices can be used in quicksand rescue?

10. What are the sides of a ladder called?

11. What is the rule regarding tidal flow?

12. Tie a bowline in a piece of string or rope with your eyes shut!

Answers on p. 212.

Safety at sporting events

Certain sporting events require the presence of first-aiders, paramedics and doctors at the site before the event can start. The organisers may approach individuals to provide this cover on a private basis. By agreeing to attend you accept a certain responsibility for the care of both spectators and competitors alike. Two major disasters at football stadiums in the UK (the Bradford fire and the Hillsborough disaster) have led to documents that clearly define the level of medical, ambulance and first aid provision expected at stadium events. These levels of provision may be assumed to apply at all large public gatherings. Furthermore, individual sporting bodies often have their own specific requirements. There is no defence against negligence by saying you didn't realise the extent of the commitment you had taken on. You will be expected to be properly equipped and experienced enough to provide the appropriate level of care. You will be expected to understand the principles of major incident management and your role within the major incident plan, and, in addition, you will be expected to be conversant with all relevant safety procedures and your powers and responsibilities to the sport as a whole.

If you find yourself at the event and the support promised by the event organisers is not to the required standard, you should refuse to stay. If you are the only doctor at the event and by regulation the event cannot then be held, the organisers could face many thousands of pounds loss and will apply considerable pressure on you, and you could face legal action for damages. This is not a commitment that should be made by a quick phone call during a coffee break – ensure that the organiser gives you all necessary details in writing. Check who will be working with you and speak to them, find out what regulations apply, and find out who is responsible for supplying equipment so that you can check the level of provision before the day.

It will be seen that the responsibility for medical care at a sporting event clearly rests with the most senior person appointed to provide that care, and this is not a role to be assumed lightly.

MOTOR SPORT SAFETY

The level of personal protective equipment required is exactly the same as for a road traffic accident, because that is exactly what you may need to deal with. Take ample food and non-alcoholic drink with you. It doesn't matter that the organiser says that the food will be provided, don't believe it till you've swallowed it. You should also remember your sun protection cream, as you can burn even on an overcast day if you are outside for 8–9 hours.

Race circuits

On arrival at the course find out where the marshals are signing on. Sign on as present and locate the rest of the medical provision. Find out where you will be working, how to get there, where it is safe to park up and what time you should be on post.

The person in overall charge is the Clerk of the Course. The clerk is responsible for the running of the meeting, the organisation, safety and judicial decisions. There are also usually three stewards at any meeting (two club stewards and a steward from the Motor Sports Association). The MSA steward has to be satisfied it is safe to run the meeting before it can start. The Clerk of the Course is based in race control, which handles radio and telephone communications to marshals' posts, emergency vehicles, scrutineers, time-keepers, etc. Marshals' posts are located around the circuit and will normally be manned by an observer, up to three flag marshals, an incident officer, and a team of fire marshals, course marshals and trainees.

Let the incident marshals secure the scene before you get involved as they will be more experienced in dealing with the incident. One of the marshals will signal the post if medical aid is required. There are five authorised hand signals (Fig. 14.1). Three are used to request assistance and two indicate safety to cross the track. They should be made clearly and be maintained until the observer acknowledges the signal by repeating it. If you are called to the incident, then use the safest route to the incident, only stepping on the track when absolutely necessary, and always looking in the direction of oncoming vehicles. If you hear a whistle, look to see what is happening and act accordingly.

If there is any incident the flag marshal will immediately display a waved yellow flag to the drivers. The observer post proceeding will display a fixed yellow flag and the one after the incident a green flag. The stationary yellow means 'slow sufficiently to give full control of the car and do not overtake'. A waved yellow means 'slow down, be prepared for evasive action and stop if necessary'. The green flag shows the hazard and the ban on overtaking is over.

Yellow flags are also displayed if a serious incident is being dealt with that requires the use of a pace or safety car. Because modern race cars

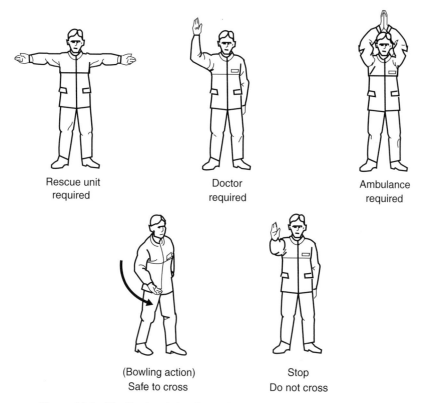

Rescue unit
required

Doctor
required

Ambulance
required

(Bowling action)
Safe to cross

Stop
Do not cross

Figure 14.1   The five hand signals used by marshals at a motor race circuit.

cannot be stopped and then restarted in the same way as a street car, every effort is made to avoid stopping the race. If necessary a pace car is introduced onto the circuit and the other vehicles follow behind. The pace car will lead the cars through a clear route at the side of the incident until it has been cleared and then turn its lights off to indicate it will leave the circuit on the next lap, allowing the race to resume. If the race must be stopped, the red flag is used. If the red flag is seen at a preceding or following post the red flag is displayed at that post, thus red flags sweep round the circuit in both directions from the point it was first displayed. A white flag is displayed if there is a slow-moving vehicle such as an ambulance or rescue vehicle in that sector.

Racing cars tend to be better protected against fire than the average street car. They often have on-board fire extinguishers and clearly marked fuel cut-off and battery cut-off switches. Methanol is sometimes used as the fuel, so it is worth remembering the flame is invisible, and Alcoseal foam is preferred. Fire marshals will fight a fire in a team of four. They will aim on approaching from upwind. Two marshals will use dry powder for the rapid knock-down effect and two will follow up with foam to prevent reignition.

Rally events

There are three main types of rallying that take place in the UK. These are the multi-venue stage rally, which involves a series of competitive stages at different locations; the multi-use single venue rally, which allows several different combinations of conditions at one location; and road rallies, which are held on public roads (often at night) and where the speed limit has to be adhered to. Obviously the last type presents a lower risk than the first two.

Rally stages may be crossed by cyclists, motor cyclists and horse riders. The marshals have a responsibility to inform everyone of the danger but cannot prevent the public from using footpaths or tracks unless they have been officially closed.

Before the race you should be supplied with a location to go to. This may be an Ordnance Survey (O.S.) map reference. You should also have instructions on how to get to the location. Follow these instructions because short cuts may well have been blocked by the police. Allow yourself plenty of time to get there. The 'stage entry' is where you leave the main road, and the 'stage start' is the location where you usually sign on and get allocated to a post by the stage commander. If it is a multi-use single venue rally, you should ensure you are issued with a stage diagram so that you know which tracks and roads are used at any given time.

A number of official cars may go through a stage before the first competitive car. They are not meant to drive at competitive speeds but some of them may do so and serious accidents have occurred in the past. You need to be prepared from the outset. The marshals' manual (Rae R: A pocket guide to marshalling) actually gives directions for righting an overturned car but clearly states that the person dealing with the casualty 'calls the shots'. The decision is affected by many factors such as the condition of the casualty, the type and availability of rescue equipment and the personnel available.

Once the course closing car has passed you may leave the area, following the direction taken during the event, or by using roads not included in the event unless express permission has been gained to go 'WD' (wrong direction).

Speed events – hill climbs and sprints

The same basic principles apply as in circuit racing except that the event is usually stopped if there is an incident and generally only a red flag is used. A whistle may be used with the flag to attract the attention of the next flag marshal. Methanol is frequently used as a fuel on hill climbs and sprints.

HORSE EVENTS

The Jockey Club lay down stringent requirements for the provision of medical services. These are to be found in a document called the *Jockey Club General Instructions* No. 11 (JCGI 11; Jockey Club 1999). Before any doctor, paramedic or first-aider undertakes to work at a race course they would be advised to read this.

Personal protective equipment primarily consists of good weatherproof clothing. The minimum requirement for a doctor is an armband saying 'DOCTOR' with a green-chequered border. Boots with toe protection are advised.

Unlike a motor race event, a horse race cannot be stopped once the horses are past the 'false start' flag. It is not uncommon for horses not to stop even when there is a false start. Once the horses have started running it is difficult and dangerous to stop them. It is also effectively impossible to let them run off the course, as it has to be entirely surrounded by barrier fencing. As a race spreads out there may be barely a couple of minutes between the passing of horses. If injuries occur at fences, which they often do, it is possible to 'dolly' the fence. Fence dolling is to take the fence out of the circuit. Marshals will deploy black and white chequered flags, traffic bollards across the fence approach, and a sign on top of the fence (Fig. 14.2). The sign displays two orange circles and a chevron indicating the direction to pass the fence. The riders will try to divert horses from jumping the fence and direct them to the side. However, as said previously, horses can fail to respond to the jockey and no absolute guarantee of safety can be assured. If attending to a fallen rider on the course a high degree of awareness must be kept at all times. A horse will try to avoid someone on the ground, but this is not possible if the horse is landing from a jump, and obviously someone can be clipped by a hoof. Serious injuries can be sustained if this occurs and the only sensible advice must be to follow the 1–2–3 of safety. You will be of no use to the rider if you become injured yourself.

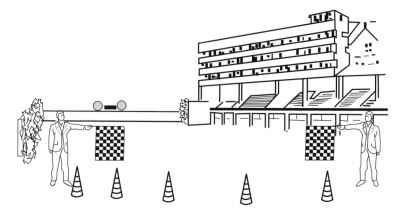

Figure 14.2   A 'dolled' fence.

Self-test questions for Chapter 14

1. Who is responsible for the quality of medical care at a sporting event?

2. Who is in charge of a motor race circuit event?

3. What flag is displayed if an incident occurs within a marshal post sector?

4. A fire marshal faces the observer post standing with his arms outstretched. What is he doing?

5. How do you 'dolly' a fence?

Answers on p. 213.

15

When people affect safety

VIOLENT PATIENTS AND BYSTANDERS

Patients may be violent for a variety of reasons. They may have psychiatric problems such as paranoia or dementia. They may have disturbed levels of consciousness due to drugs, alcohol, mental illness, hypoglycaemia, hypoxia or head injury. They may not understand what is happening, or may be hysterical with fear. They may face major loss or criminal proceedings if their plans are foiled. The fact is that 67% of ambulance personnel and 13% of general practitioners surveyed recently had suffered physical assault.

Violent behaviour may come after clear warning signs, or, less commonly, may occur without any prior warning. Often when there is a violent episode the warning signs have been ignored. Ambulance personnel generally receive little training in how to approach an incident in a manner that will give them the greatest chance of a safe outcome from a violent situation. Doctors generally receive no training unless they deliberately seek it out.

The American emergency services are well used to approaching an incident scene in a manner that will minimise risk. This is done routinely and is designed to keep the element of surprise on the side of the responder. In the UK there is now an awareness of the need for caution, although people watching emergency personnel approach a building or a car will be largely unaware of the systematic checks that are being made during the approach.

Emergency personnel will, however, be practising risk assessment and minimising potential harm. No longer can emergency service personnel rush in to a scene. When responding to a stabbing you may be thinking of tension pneumothorax, arterial blood loss and the need for an air ambulance. You should be thinking, 'Where is the assailant? Is the scene secure? Is the scene safe to enter?' The police should be summoned if there is the risk of violence.

Coded radio signals may be part of an established protocol for the management of violence. Unfortunately there is no universal radio code. Some services use 'Message 13', others use 'Code 10–7' or 'Message 66'; there are also services that use 'Code 9'. Controllers must be responsive to the needs of the crew. It is not uncommon to hear controllers asking for details of the situation to give to the police and demonstrating a reluctance to press the panic button when it is apparent from the guarded tones the crew are using that they fear saying more in the individual's earshot. There is an argument for a simple message that conveys a little more information. The addition of a colour would indicate which service was required, and the 1–2–3 of safety could be utilised so that a 'Message 13 Blue 1' would mean, 'I require immediate police presence because I am in danger', whereas 'Message 13 Red 3' would mean, 'I need an immediate fire service response because the life of the casualty is in danger'.

Ambulance crews are frequently called to residential areas to assist a person injured in an assault or a domestic dispute, and the experienced crew will automatically exercise some caution; but these are not the only ones that can lead to danger. Be suspicious of any call that involves 'severe bleeding'. An 'attempted suicide' could end up with you being the victim of a murder. Most of all, do not expect to see friendly faces to greet you when you arrive at a 'nature unknown' call. If the caller is too hysterical to provide complete information to the telephonist, the controller should share this information with the crew. Until you know the reason for the hysteria, you must proceed with caution.

ARRIVING ON SCENE TO A BUILDING

If the emergency crew are to keep the situation under their control they need to enter the scene in such a manner as to allow a controlled assessment. To pull up in front of a house with blue lights flashing and to jump from the vehicle with equipment in both hands immediately makes the crew a target for any aggression. If at all possible the lights and horns should not be used after entering the immediate neighbourhood to avoid losing the element of surprise, and to avoid attracting a crowd. If the ambulance is stopped directly in front of a building the occupants can watch your every move and still remain unseen. Parking spaces can be limited but ideally the crew should pull past the residence, allowing observation of the house from three sides. The vehicle should be parked just beyond an imaginary line running 45° from the edge of the house. Always park to escape with a direct route, rather than needing to turn the vehicle first. Always turn off the headlights before the attendant walks towards the building if there is the risk that they will make a silhouette. When approaching a multistorey building scan the windows, balconies and roof line for signs of an ambush. If you need to walk under windows or balconies to enter a building, wear your helmet, and once the building has been scanned, do not look up again to prevent a falling object striking you in the face.

If the block of flats has an entry phone system it is recommended that you should ring any doorbell except the correct one to maintain the element of surprise. If it has been possible to park at an angle to the house it should be approached from an angle if possible. Both crew members should approach the building together as the attendant will establish contact with the casualty while his or her colleague will continue to assess the safety situation. Listen to what you can hear from the outside, look for evidence of violence, assess the number of voices heard. If at any time danger seems apparent then back away from the house towards the ambulance. Do not turn your back, keep the source of your anxiety in sight. Call your control, explain the problem and move to a position of safety to await a police attendance.

Most front doors open inwards. By standing to the lock side of the door the occupant will have to open the door to see you, whereas if you stand near the hinge they will see you from opening the door only a crack (Fig. 15.1). Use the the ability to see into the building to your advantage. Is the person behaving appropriately? Does his or her clothing suggest a recent struggle? Is the person carrying a potential weapon? Look at the room, and also between door and the frame on the hinge side to see if someone is hiding behind the door.

When the incident is at a block of flats it may not be possible to stand to the side of the door because of the way the circulation space is designed. One option is to knock on the door and then withdraw quickly to the staircase and announce yourself from there. Wait until the door is opened and the resident behaves appropriately before entering.

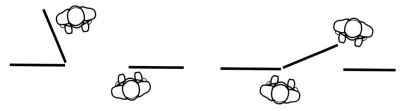

Figure 15.1   Standing at the lock side of a door increases your view when the door is opened.

Ideally emergency service personnel would have access to a key allowing the lift to be put to the firefighter's service. Alternatively you may consider using a snatch bag or piece of equipment to keep the door open. The lift should be held on the floor of the emergency until you are ready to descend. Look for the stairwell and check the door can be opened. The stairs may be needed as a secondary escape route. If the door to the flat is open on your arrival do not go inside without permission. Knock on the door, announce who you are, and wait for someone to come to the door before moving in front of the door way. If they call 'come in' without coming to the door, be wary. Ask them if they can step outside to talk to you before you enter. If they cannot, find out why. You should have already been informed if they are providing cardio-pulmonary resuscitation (CPR) or telephone first aid. If they cannot give a good reason, consider withdrawing until you have police support. If the person claims to be alone and too ill or injured to come to the door, proceed with caution.

PROCEDURE ONCE INSIDE THE BUILDING

When entering any room move briskly through the doorway until you are in the room. Silhouetted in the doorway you are in what has been termed the 'kill zone' (Fig. 15.2). You are in a position that an assailant knows you will occupy, and will be concentrating on, while you suddenly have a wide angle of visual data to assimilate before you identify any risk. Scan the room for risks in the form of potential assailants and potential weapons.

Ask the occupants to show you where the patient is to be found. Let them lead you to the patient. They will be providing you with the quickest route to the casualty and they will be protecting you from attack. The

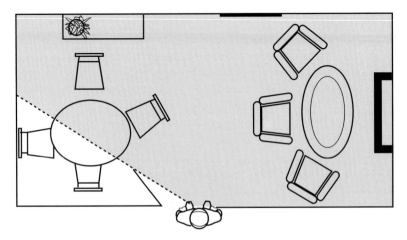

Figure 15.2 Standing in the kill zone.

person who answers the door is usually known to the casualty and is less likely to be perceived as a threat than a pair of strangers.

If the victim has an injury that could have been inflicted by another person, do your very best not to let the other occupants out of your sight until you have determined who or what caused the injury. If one of the occupants starts to leave, ask him or her to assist by holding the i.v. bag, steadying the patient's legs, etc., so that you can keep the person in sight. This will reduce the possibility of the individual being the unidentified assailant and obtaining a further weapon. If the person insists on going to another room and refuses to allow you to follow, then both you and your partner should leave immediately, with the casualty if at all possible, even if unorthodox means are required. If the patient hesitates or starts to argue, leave him or her behind. Do not stop to gather your equipment; leave the house and call for the police from a safe location. Arrange to meet with the police officers and explain the situation before they enter the building. They need to know the layout, the number of people present, what caused you to leave and the condition of the casualty if he or she was left behind. If one crew member feels the need to leave, then both should leave. You should document that:

- The behaviour of the people present led you to believe you were in danger.
- You acted for your own safety.
- You did not wait to pack your equipment before leaving.
- All non-police personnel left at the same time.
- You did not leave the scene, only the danger area.
- The police were called as an emergency.
- You returned to the casualty as soon as the situation was safe.

If there are potential weapons in the room, try to move them from the reach of the casualty and the occupants by 'casually' involving them in the process of laying out your equipment. Bear in mind that guns and knives may have fingerprint evidence that could be destroyed by incautious handling. Ideally, move the casualty away from the weapon, using the need for light or space as an excuse. If you must move the weapon remember where it originally lay and inform the police officer attending the incident.

Most ambulance crews turning up to a domestic disturbance in progress will have the sense to await the arrival of the police before entering the building. Often, however, the sight of blood and the shock of injury calms the dispute, only for it to flare again as each party tries to win the allegiance and sympathy of the emergency personnel. If this happens, separate the fighting parties as quickly as possible, but never stand between them. You can only have your attention on one of two potential assailants at a time, and are likely to be attacked by both.

The crew should work as a team, each taking one protagonist and, using voice commands, eye contact and body language, should manipulate the people to turn away from each other until they are back to back. Once they lose sight of each other they will tend to quieten down.

CONTROL TECHNIQUES

Speech can provide the most effective means of keeping out of trouble. Your pressure of speech, your tone and the words you say can affect the behaviour of the protagonists. You are trying to convey that you respect each of them as individuals, that you are independent in the quarrel, and that you expect them to behave in a civilised manner while you do your job.

To achieve these aims you should always address the individuals as 'Sir' or 'Ma'am', use 'please' and 'thank you', and ask permission before taking any action that could be seen as an invasion of personal space. Do not forget to explain your actions to the individual.

People who are arguing are usually talking or shouting at each other rather than listening to each other. They are not using the logical part of their personality but are coming out with previously learnt attitudes or emotions. Asking a question clearly relevant to the casualty's care but on a subject unrelated to the argument in hand forces the individual to stop behaving attitudinally or emotionally and reply with a logical answer. A series of questions of this type often switches the person back into logical behaviour.

If the crew members take separate protagonists and establish eye contact and introduce themselves and make appropriate enquiries, then, by maintaining eye contact and continued speech, it is possible to move slowly in a circular direction to turn the individuals away from each other. There are, however, certain key points to the procedure. Do not turn an individual so that they block your exit. Do not lose sight of your partner and glance towards the individual he or she is interviewing to ensure there are no weapons being hidden that may be used. If you see a weapon, warn your partner by a prearranged code word such as calling him or her by an abbreviated name not normally used. The use of tables and sofas as a physical barrier between parties should be considered as the individuals are re-positioned.

The best position to adopt when talking to people involved in a dispute is the 'interview stance'. You should stand approximately an arm's length away from the person with your body at a 45° angle, with the non-dominant foot forward. Have your feet a shoulder width apart, with the weight mainly on the rear foot. The knees should be just less than locked fully extended. Keep your clip board or response bag in your non-dominant hand to use as a shield if required. This position appears innocuous but allows you to step back rapidly out of range and shield yourself. If the clipboard or bag is grabbed, let them have it and make your escape.

There are a variety of defensive moves that can be applied if you are grabbed or attacked. It is not the remit of this text to teach these techniques, as they are best demonstrated. Seek instruction from a police officer if you feel that you may need to use such methods.

ENTERING BARS AND CLUBS

Begin to consider the problem as soon as the call is received. Does the establishment have a reputation for trouble? Is the incident due to illness, accident or assault? If an assault, is the assailant still on the premises? Has the scene been secured by police or doormen? Are the police responding, and what is their ETA, (estimated time of arrival)? Do not enter a building unsupported unless you know you will be able to maintain radio communications from inside. Do not enter alone; always go as a pair. Always confirm with control that the police have been notified and are responding.

Entering a dimly lit establishment before you become dark adapted places you at risk. To partially compensate for subdued lighting you can try keeping your dominant eye closed from leaving the vehicle until you are inside the building. This eye will be partially dark adapted and will assist you peering into the dimness. Your peripheral vision adapts more quickly than central vision, so keep your eyes moving around the room, bringing areas of interest into off-centre view.

Again, do not pause in the kill zone, particularly with a light behind you. Step to the side of the door and keep the wall close behind you. Assess the room so that you can decide to proceed or withdraw to await police support. If you feel the need to withdraw, tell your colleague, 'We will need the stretcher straight away' – and both withdraw. The doormen or barman will usually be the most co-operative, and the most sober. While one crew member tends to the patient, the other should monitor the room and watch his or her partner's back, unless door staff are prepared to maintain this degree of protection. Be aware of the potential for a situation to deteriorate. Evacuation should be more 'scoop and run' than 'stay and play'.

ARRIVING ON SCENE TO A VEHICLE

Road traffic accidents have their own risks, and occasionally 'road rage' can have continued as an assault after the incident, but these are not the only occasions when ambulances are called to vehicles. From car bombs to ambushes, certain features should give rise to caution.

- You arrive at the scene with blue lights and two-tone horn. Heads are visible in the vehicle, but nobody turns round or moves.
- You arrive at the scene of a cardiac arrest in a car. The car is neatly parked with no visible occupants.

- As you stop your vehicle all the occupants of the car get out and start to walk towards you.
- The driver adjusts the rear or side view mirror and watches your every move.
- The vehicle and the occupants appear out of place for the neighbourhood.
- Weapons are seen lying in the street.
- You enter a potential ambush zone.
- You have a gut feeling.

All these situations are examples of abnormal behaviour. They do not 'add up'. You should withdraw and await the arrival of the police to secure the scene.

The ambulance should be parked at least 5 metres behind the vehicle, on a 10° angle and the wheels turned out towards the road to facilitate a rapid withdrawal. In this position the rear beacons will still be in line with traffic to provide security, and the wheels will propel the vehicle away from the incident if it is shunted, but also the wheels will act as physical protection if firearms are used.

Before you leave the vehicle you should note the licence number, colour and make of the car on a pad and leave it beside the radio in the vehicle. At night the headlights should be put on full beam to illuminate the interior of the vehicle and its immediate perimeter. If the driver has a spotlight or quartz halogen torch, then this should be shone at the rear view mirror. This will effectively prevent the occupants seeing the approach of the attendant to the car. The ambulance cab courtesy light should be switched so that it remains off when the door is opened.

You should dismount with the snatch bag and quietly close the door. Your torch should be off and used only when needed, to minimise identifying yourself as a target. When using the torch it should be held away from the body. You should walk behind your own vehicle to avoid being caught in its lights, and pause at the driver's door to check that no untoward action has occurred while you were passing behind the ambulance.

If all appears well, then progress from the driver's door to the rear of the car as quickly and quietly as possible. Put the snatch bag on the ground near the vehicle boot, but not where it could trip you if you have to run for your life. Lightly place your hand on the boot lid to ensure that it is secure. This will not move the vehicle but will indicate if someone could be hiding inside. If the boot lid feels higher, or movement is felt from within the boot, slam the lid to prevent the occupant from exiting without lifting it first. Be constantly aware for a 'click' that might indicate that the driver has released the boot catch from inside the car. If you hear it you should retreat immediately.

Stand sideways to the vehicle and keep belly-in to the car. This not only minimises your presentation as a target to the occupants, but also gives you maximum protection from passing vehicles. Stop alongside the C post and look in the rear and side windows, notice the number of occupants and particularly where their hands are. Try to see what items are on the seats and the floor. Look for weapons. If you see a knife or a gun, retreat to a safe area and call the police.

If the rear seat is occupied do not pass the C post, but if all appears satisfactory move forward to the B post. Do not move further forwards as you will be moving into the kill zone. Tap on the window and announce, 'Ambulance Service, do you need help?'

Do not reach into the car for any reason as the driver could grab your arm and pull you into the car or against the roof. He could then trap you with the window, stab you or even drive off. Once you have established the need for medical care check the vehicle is in neutral and the brake is on, and then signal for your driver to bring any necessary equipment forward.

Approaches to vans with sliding side doors should be made on the passenger side, but walk forwards until 45° forward of the A post, keeping at least 3–5 metres away from the side door. This procedure keeps you away from the possibility of an occupant leaping from the side door to attack you.

If it is essential to park facing the vehicle in question, then effectively combine the procedure for cars and vans. Exit, pass around the rear of your vehicle, check with the driver, then walk forwards staying 3–5 metres away from the car until you are at 45° to the rear of the C post. Then continue the approach as before.

TRANSPORTING THE SUSPECT CASUALTY

It is not uncommon for an ambulance crew to be expected to transport a casualty who has been violent, or who is irrational and may become violent. The worst scenario is an unrestrained casualty who produces a previously concealed weapon while the attendant is alone with the individual in the vehicle saloon during a journey to hospital. Potentially violent casualties should not be transported by ambulance unless the danger to their health precludes use of police transport.

The casualty should be given a body search in the guise of a secondary survey, and then secured to a long board 'for the protection of their spine'. A 'spider's web' strapping is more effective than buckles and straps. Do not allow the casualty access to any handbag, purse, briefcase or other hiding place for a concealed weapon during transport.

If receiving a patient from a prison or police station, then you should ask the officer in charge to confirm the casualty has been searched for contraband. Record any injuries that they may have, as it is not uncommon for injuries to be self-inflicted before the doctor examines them, and these to be attributed to the custody staff.

TAKING COVER

It is important to recognise the difference between structures that offer protection against projectiles and those that offer concealment only. The uninitiated often think that if they can't see the assailant, then the assailant can't see them. Hiding behind an ambulance is of limited value as the glass fibre body offers little protection against a high-velocity round. Furthermore the angle of incidence is not the same as the angle of reflection when it comes to bullets. The bullet deforms as it hits the ground and the ricochet is therefore angled much closer to the ground. At least one ambulance worker has been killed by the marksman deliberately firing on the ground in front of the ambulance (Fig. 15.3).

The wheels and engine block provide the greatest cover from a vehicle. A lamp post will not give complete cover and you will risk being shot in the arm, knee or shoulder. Whenever possible choose cover that allows you to stand. If trapped for an extended period it is the most comfortable and versatile position, allowing you to shift your weight without revealing yourself. It also leaves you ready to change your location rapidly if the need arises. Do not change location just for the sake of doing so. Only move if it takes you further from the danger and you can move without revealing yourself. If you are forced into moving then do not run in a direct line from the gunman's position, as this allows a careful aim to be made – rather run in a zigzag pattern.

Items inside a building can give you cover provided they are substantial enough. A refrigerator will provide cover but a sofa or plasterboard wall will not. If concealment is the only option available, then be aware of its limitations.

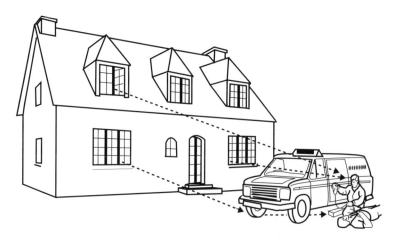

Figure 15.3 Lines of fire open to the marksman.

Street lighting can silhouette you or can cast your shadow where it can be seen. People can be accurately located from making too much sound and your high-visibility clothing makes concealment difficult. Consider turning it inside out.

HOSTAGE SITUATIONS

Hostage situations do not frequently involve the ambulance service. Doctors have been held hostage on several occasions recently, but the situations do occur regularly. The average incident lasts between 4 and 5 hours. Provided you do not panic, you have in excess of a 95% chance of escaping physically unscathed. Try to anticipate the feelings and the actions of the hostage-taker and those of the police.

Hostage-takers are loosely classified as 'crazy, criminal or crusading'. People with mental illness account for half of the hostage incidents. They may see you as someone who is against them because you are: (a) trying to get them into hospital, or (b) trying to get someone they have injured into hospital. The major mental illnesses involved in hostage-taking are schizophrenia, severe depression, inadequate personality and psychopathic personality. Criminals usually take hostages from people who are present at a crime when something goes wrong. Crusaders are terrorists, and the group least likely to be encountered. Terrorist activities are well planned and carefully executed and so your value to their goal is probably limited.

There are six stages to a hostage situation, but some of them may be omitted in any particular circumstance.

Surveillance stage

This is the stage that is characteristic of the crusader hostage-taker, though it may be used by criminal hostage-takers if the intent is to use the victim for monetary gain. It involves detailed research of the intended hostage's behaviour to minimise the risk of the action going wrong.

Capture stage

When an emergency service worker is taken hostage both parties are likely to be as surprised as each other. The mentally disturbed and the criminal rarely plan to take uniformed individuals as hostages, and if it happens it is usually to use them as a medium for negotiation or as a shield for their escape.

The hostage-taker will be very anxious, having lost control of the situation. This is the most dangerous moment of the situation; you must assume that the individual will use his or her weapon if you do not immediately follow instructions. You should not attempt to escape. If the action fails your new relationship with your captor will be even worse. You must remain calm and control your anger.

Transport stage

You may be transported from where you were taken hostage to a place where your captor feels more secure. This may only be across the room, or may be to another part of the building. If transport occurs shortly after capture the individual will still be very agitated. Commands will be harsh, and if you move too slowly you may well be physically harmed. You may be tied, gagged and blindfolded and this will distort your perceptions. Panic will try to set in. If faced with this situation try to concentrate on where you are being taken. Use your perception of movement, and your senses of hearing and smell to try to build up a picture of where you are going. This information will be of value later. Concentrating on it now will help take your mind off your fear.

Holding stage

The situation has by now usually calmed a little, the police are usually on the scene and they are negotiating for your release. Accept that you have no control whatsoever over when you will be freed. Do not do anything that will attract unwanted attention. The sole reason you are alive is because you are a bargaining tool. Do not pressure them or agitate them, particularly female hostage-takers, as they are usually easy to anger and prone to using violence. You should try to find a middle ground between cowardice and heroism. You do not want to stand out. You may need to ask for food or permission to sleep or use the toilet. Remember to be courteous. If offered food or the opportunity to use the toilet, accept the offer graciously. You will not necessarily get what you want in food, or privacy in using the toilet. Try to accept this.

Movement stage

If the incident is protracted then there may well be a further relocation. This usually only can take place if the police have not located and surrounded your position. Be very wary of trying the boy scout trick of leaving clues behind. If your captors spot them then you may well be killed as a warning to other hostages and as an indication that their demands must be met by the authorities.

Resolution

Whenever possible the police negotiators will wait until the holding stage and the reduction in emotional levels before establishing contact with your captors. They will be gathering information about the hostages and their captors during this waiting period. When contact is made the negotiators will try to do it by telephone. Ultimately the situation will be resolved by your release or by an assault from an armed response team. Stay away from doors and windows. If there is a rescue bid stun grenades may well be used. If there is an assault on the position then you should lie on the floor and place your hands on your head. Remain in that position until your rescuers tell you to move. Expect to be treated as a suspect. Follow your rescuers' instructions completely. There will be plenty of opportunity to thank your rescuers after the scene has been declared safe.

CIVIL DISTURBANCE

In times past, a local magistrate would literally read the Riot Act to the crowd and, if they did not disperse, the militia would exert whatever force was necessary to stop civil disturbance. Policing has changed somewhat since then. A civil disorder is defined as any situation in which the conduct of individuals will, in the opinion of the police service, require special arrangements to deal with it and its consequences.

The police must be seen as the emergency service that has overall authority during periods of civil disturbance. The role of ambulance crews and immediate care doctors is always to provide care to the sick and injured and evacuate them to hospital. To achieve this personnel should have trained with the police to ensure a common working format. Plans vary from region to region but the common features are that ambulance and medical personnel work behind police lines in a rescue role. Their responsibility is to work in conjunction with the police to extricate casualties and convey them to safety. They are expected to make every effort not only to maintain but also to clearly demonstrate neutrality.

When faced with civil disturbance personal protective equipment acquires a new importance. The standard ambulance helmet to the original Pacific design gives no protection to the neck and acid or petrol that strikes the top of the helmet will flow behind the visor when it is down. The new Pacific helmet and the Gallet helmet give better protection in this respect. The flammability of the normal tunic has already been discussed. It is far more important that suits are made of fire- and acid-resistant material such as Nomax. Firefighter gloves and boots are recommended. SP Services have recently started selling lightweight Kevlar body armour similar to that worn by the police. This can prevent knife and bullet penetration. There is an argument that wearing body armour incites hostility. Decisions to purchase such equipment need to be made after consultation with police and trades unions, and taken after a formal risk assessment. An important consideration must be that supplies may not be available at times of civil disturbance. There are several grades of body armour and obviously the better the grade, the more cumbersome it is to wear. It is necessary that personal protective equipment is appropriate to the risk, and therefore will depend upon the type of weapons in use in that locality.

Team working and good communications are essential if personal safety is to be ensured. If instructed to evacuate an area by the police, then that order must be obeyed immediately or serious injury could result.

The *Ambulance Service Basic Training Manual* (Institute of Health Service Development, 1999) gives three types of incident: the standing disorder, the running disorder and the ambush.

Standing disorder

When a crowd is contained, such as with a protest outside an embassy or at a pop concert, the ambulance service can deploy small teams, usually of three personnel, at a safe distance behind police lines, to assist in the care of casualties. The police provide their own advanced trained first-aiders to deal with wounded in a 'hot' zone. Only life-saving procedures are applied before the person is evacuated to an ambulance. Delay in treating one casualty may prevent the evacuation of another, or lead to further injuries because the police cannot fall back as they are protecting a fallen comrade. Personnel must be aware that the situation can change rapidly and previously safe areas may need urgent evacuation. Vehicles must therefore always be in such a condition as to allow rapid retreat. Park facing the escape route; do not unload equipment not in use. Ensure the battery does not become flattened from use of the saloon lights, and do not allow one vehicle to obstruct the escape route of others.

You must not allow ambulances or medical vehicles to be used to deploy police. Such an action is directly contrary to the principle of neutrality, though if a safe area is being overrun it is permitted to allow police officers to escape in a vehicle if this is the only way to ensure their safety. When attending incidents at night vehicles should travel with saloon lights on to clearly show that police are not occupying the vehicle.

Mob violence is totally unpredictable. Doctors, ambulance crews and their vehicles might be thought by some as travelling with a freedom similar to that of the Red Cross. That is not necessarily the case. The direction violence takes depends on a variety of factors. If the cause of the disturbance is perceived to be against 'anyone in authority' or if rumour suggests the ambulance service has not been neutral, or if alcohol has been freely consumed, or professional agitators have been at work, the wearing of a green uniform will make no difference whatsoever. Dramatic acts where one person turns back a mob is the stuff of films, and cannot be relied upon to work in real life.

Running disorder

In certain situations, particularly when whole neighbourhoods are in a state of agitation, the police will try to prevent the formation of large groups. This can result in small groups of young people carrying out a series of 'hit and run' attacks. A vehicle may be required to attend an emergency in the community. It may be possible to organise escort by respected community leaders to protect a vehicle and its crew. A crew of four should attend when possible. This allows two crew to evacuate the casualty to the ambulance rapidly while the rear doors are kept fully open and secured with a look-out and guard in the back. The engine is kept running with a driver in the driving seat and the cab doors locked. As soon as the patient is on board the vehicle should leave the scene. Normal care procedures are undertaken in transit.

Ambush

The *Ambulance Service Basic Training Manual* states that where there is a potential for an ambush to occur vehicles will normally be escorted by the police. This takes little account of the fact that a successful ambush uses the element of surprise, and will therefore probably occur when that provision has not been made.

The reasons for ambush may be theft, vandalism, hostage-taking, assault on the casualty, or to allow infiltration to secure areas by the 'Trojan horse' approach. The safety of the casualty and the crew is of paramount importance and situations may develop for which no protocol has ever been devised.

The best way of avoiding an ambush is to have a high index of suspicion. The call for the ambulance may have aroused suspicions at control and they may think the call is a hoax. An ambush is likely to occur in an area that is remote but it will be an urban or inner city environment. It will probably be an area where it is difficult to escape, a cul-de-sac for example. Crews should routinely reverse into and block a cul-de-sac. There may be a young adult to lead the crew away 'to the emergency' or there may be no-one in sight. The body language of the person may seem strange. You may see a vehicle moving to block your escape route, but by the time this is noticed it is getting too late to control the situation. The most important action if you think you might be at risk of ambush is to inform control. If you can retreat to an area where your options for escape are increased, then do so. If you can lock yourself in the vehicle, do so – windows may be smashed or doors forced, but this limits the value of the vehicle as a Trojan horse. It also maximises the protection that can be afforded to any casualty. If resistance is causing an increase in frustration and help is not rapidly available, then it is wise to surrender. A body language of respectful submission and a non-confrontational attitude is the best approach in these circumstances. Follow the advice given in the section on hostages.

IMPROVISED EXPLOSIVE DEVICES

Just as in hostage situations, explosive devices can be produced by 'crazies, criminals and crusaders' but to these categories must also be added a further 'C' word – 'children'. The instructions for making home-made explosives can be easily obtained from the Internet. A 10-minute search gave me the recipe for a device I could make with household ingredients 'that packs a force equivalent to approximately half a stick of dynamite'. Generally, ambulance services are reasonably protected from the criminal and the crusader. Criminals recognise that unprovoked aggression towards ambulance personnel will not be tolerated in either the law enforcement agencies or the criminal fraternity. Crusaders are also aware that such an attack would alienate them from public sympathy, generally not something they wish to do. This just leaves the 'crazies' and the 'children'.

Unfortunately, it is becoming more common in society for people to resort to aggression when they are dissatisfied with the outcome of a life event. In the heat of an immediate care scenario it is possible for individuals to perceive that paramedics or doctors actually caused the death of a loved one rather than tried to save them. The psychiatrically unstable can become locked in the anger phase that is a natural part of grieving and then start to plot revenge. The individual will usually want 'those responsible' to suffer, and so threats and intimidation often preceed any life-endangering acts.

If threats are received they must be taken seriously and reported to the police as well as to senior officers. Written threats should be saved in their entirety with the minimum of handling to preserve any fingerprints. If the threat is an anonymous telephone call then you should make as many notes as possible while the caller is on the line. Listen to the voice (male or female), voice quality (calm or excited), accents or impediments. Try to record as accurately as possible everything said by the caller. Pay attention to background noise such as traffic, music, motors, etc. that could give a clue to the location of the caller. Pay-as-you-go mobile phones are impossible to trace to an individual, so this information is as essential as it was in the days of the mechanical exchange. Finally, check to see whether the number was recorded on the automatic number recording service (1471) – it's unlikely, but stranger things have happened.

If you believe yourself to be at risk from aggression, then it is important that you gain, and take the advice of, the police at a suitably senior level. Sometimes junior officers can be dismissive of what sounds to be 'playing scared', but this attitude should not be accepted and representation to your employers or the emergency service representative on the immediate care scheme committee will usually result in an appropriate response. You should not try to conceal the risk from your family or your fellow workers; they may be at risk as well, either because the perpetrator wishes to cause you anguish by hurting them, or they may accidentally be exposed to a threat designed for you.

Although the appearance of letter bombs varies widely there are some characteristics that tend to show up repeatedly. Because bombers do not want to face a post office counter clerk, parcels often have excess postage, or they have been delivered by hand and have no postage or unfranked stamps on them. They will be unexpected parcels, without a return address or a fictitious address. They often have 'Personal', 'Private', 'Fragile – Handle with Care' or 'Rush – Urgent Package' on them. The label may be done in Letraset, or written with a distorted handwriting. There may be excessive use of Sellotape and perhaps string. Letter bombs may feel rigid, appear uneven or lopsided in weight. The postmark may be different from the return address. The parcel may have protruding wire, aluminium foil, oil stains or even emit a peculiar odour. If suspected the item should be isolated and the immediate area evacuated for 50 metres. Do not put it in water or confine the space around it. If possible open windows in the immediate area.

The situation with children is different. The explosive is usually made for fun, and malice is not intended. Unfortunately, because the destructive potential is often poorly understood, the explosive may be in a highly unstable condition when it is found. The child is aware that he or she has done something for which there could be punishment and will often fail to declare the risk. The most common explosives are those made using 'weed-killer formulas'. They are unstable, and have characteristics similar to gunpowder in that the real explosive potential is only exhibited when confined. An unconfined quantity of this type of material can still cause extensive damage to hands and face if it detonates nearby. It is the material used to make pipe bombs and nail bombs, so the presence of these materials with a male between 10 and 20 years of age who has sustained burn or blast injury should arouse extreme suspicion. Evacuate the area with the casualty as soon as the risk is suspected, but leave any bags, satchels, etc. untouched at scene. Do not move anything if it can be avoided, do not allow people to smoke, do not use oxygen, and do not use your radio until you are at least 50 metres away from the suspected device. Ensure the police secure the scene and are aware of the danger.

Self-test questions for Chapter 15

1. You are called to a house in a run-down council estate. The call is to an elderly lady who has fallen down stairs. Control has warned you that the male caller, her son, became abusive when the dispatcher tried to talk him through telephone aid. There is a car with flat tyres in the delapidated garden, the rest of the house looks in similar condition. What actions do you take?

2. List some of the factors that should arouse suspicions when attending a vehicle where someone has become ill.

3. Give three reasons why traditional PPE is inadequate in situations of civil disturbance.

4. What three types of civil disturbance are considered in the *Ambulance Service Basic Training Manual*?

5. What considerations should be given to attending in support of the police at civil disorder incidents?

6. What factors would lead you to suspect a potential ambush?

7. What characteristics might make you suspect a mail bomb?

Answers on p. 214.

Training for hazardous occupations

In 1984 the Health and Safety Executive produced a document entitled *Training for Hazardous Occupations* (OP8). The purpose of the document was to consider the conflict that arises between the various pieces of legislation on health and safety and the fact that certain tasks that need to be performed are inherently dangerous.

Generally it is assumed that emergency personnel accept that they may be exposed to risks, and at an incident they will continue to work for the benefit of those who are involved. They have a right to be provided with adequate protective equipment and to be trained in its use. Furthermore, they have the right to be trained in the safest way of managing situations they may encounter in their employment.

The situation is different when it comes to training. In such circumstances the risk may only be acceptable if those undergoing the training are aware of the hazard to which they are to be exposed, fully understand why it is necessary, and appreciate the benefits gained by it.

The Health and Safety at Work Act 1974 (Department of Employment 1974) is not written in absolute terms, containing the words 'so far as is reasonably practicable'. There is therefore a judgement that needs to be made between minimising the risks emergency personnel will take with any rescue, and the risk to the public if the rescue is not undertaken.

Situations have occurred where rescues have been abandoned in favour of a much more measured recovery of a body because the officer in charge has determined that the risk to the emergency personnel outweighed the probability of finding the casualty alive. Decisions like this have been backed up by the courts. It is unforgivable for someone to lose their life in an uncontrolled and ill-considered rescue of a corpse. All emergency personnel must be prepared to review the sense of continuing with a rescue in these circumstances, but the decision will often rest heavily with the paramedic or doctor as they are the ones who decide when the life is to be despaired of.

The basic health and safety philosophy is to provide a safe environment, in which safe systems of work can occur, and finally to provide personal protective equipment as a 'longstop' against injury. This concepts of 'Safe Place', 'Safe Practice' and 'Safe Person' cannot be achieved when there is no control over the environment in which emergency personnel are working. No two incidents are identical, so precise procedures cannot be formulated, but basic principles of safety can be adapted to cover all situations.

To develop the ability to apply correctly basic safety principles and skills, regular training must be undertaken. While firefighters will generally deal with many of the environmental hazards that can occur, paramedics and doctors are increasingly needed alongside the entrapped casualty to provide the optimum casualty management. The fire service cannot be expected to render the environment totally safe before medical staff enter and, because of the nature of emergencies, cannot guarantee to spot unsafe practice by them before it has had consequences. Furthermore, ambulance crews and doctors may arrive at incidents well in advance of the fire service. Paramedics, immediate care doctors and police officers should therefore all be involved in safety training.

In training it is possible to take the necessary time to provide additional safeguards to ensure the safety of those taking part. This enables the risks that may be involved in future hazardous operations to be introduced gradually in order that safeguards can be practised that will protect rescuers at real incidents.

Training often involves exposure to environments that can cause fear. Unless these environments have been experienced and the emotions controlled before real life exposure there is a grave risk of serious harm occurring at an incident. The 'Safety at Scene' courses provide realistic training in a safe environment and are therefore ideal opportunities for emergency services to fulfil their responsibilities under the Health and Safety at Work legislation.

Manual handling techniques

In the normal workplace considerable attention can be paid to ergonomics. This is the study of how the human structure interacts with the environment around it. Heavy objects that need to be moved can be jacked or hoisted into place. Structures can be arranged to provide an optimum situation in those cases where only 'person power' will suffice. This is not the case for the emergency services, however. Despite all the best efforts at designing equipment that requires less physical force to operate, and identifying equipment that requires more than one person to lift, the very nature of rescue means emergency personnel will often be faced with moving heavy loads from difficult positions. The almost infinite variety of problems that can face rescuers means that no series of techniques can possibly cover all eventualities. The only alternative is to explain the principles of safe handling, bearing in mind the machine that will have to be used, i.e. the human body.

The human machine is extremely versatile, but this very quality also creates weaknesses within it. Furthermore there are several major design flaws that have resulted from the evolution of the machine. If the human were to be designed afresh from the drawing board, the construction would be radically different. The weakest point when considering heavy manual labour must be the design of the spine, and the greatest strength is the human brain.

SIMPLE BIOMECHANICS

There were a series of evolutionary advantages to be gained when our ancestors acquired the ability to walk erect. They could see further, reach further, and by having less surface area in direct sunlight could shed the extra heat that higher levels of brain function produced. The spine was designed for four legs, however. The human spine originally evolved as a bridge from which was suspended a chest cage and an abdominal cavity.

The curved spine gave maximum ability to extend and rotate the head, a large capacity for the lungs and a superbly strong lower spine from which to suspend the intestines. Then our ancestors ruined it by deciding to walk on two legs rather than four.

The lower limbs and pelvis effectively produce an arch on which everything else is stacked, and it is the lumbar spine that is the only rigid structure that prevents the ribs crashing onto the pelvis. The whole weight of the chest and the head, the arms and whatever they carry must be supported on the lumbar spine. Probably half the body weight is above the lumbar spine, so approximately 100 pounds (45 kg) is balanced on the three to four square inches of lumbar spine when an average man is standing erect. This is around the pressure that car tyres are inflated to. It wouldn't be too bad if the spine were as solid as a femur, but it can't be. To allow for bending, stretching and twisting the spine must be a series of separate bricks with a flexible joint between each. The discs that lie between each bony vertebra are an example of evolutionary engineering at its best. They are very like lozenge-shaped golf balls. They consist of a very thick short tube of elastic fibres, wound round and round, with a gooey soft jelly-like centre filling. The centre filling distributes the load equally onto the tissues that contain it.

When lifting a load the weight is passed on to the lumbar spine. A 14-stone (88 kg) paramedic is already putting 100 pounds onto his lumbar spine, but if he then tries to lift one end of a stretcher with a 14-stone man on he will add another 100 pounds and the weight of half a stretcher. The muscles surrounding the vertebrae pull like guy-ropes to ensure the bones stay stacked in alignment. It only requires a sudden unexpected movement for a muscle to tear as it tries desperately to stabilise the load. If the load is carried at arm's length the arm acts as a lever on the intervertebral disc and increases the load applied by up to five times.

As the years pass the elastic fibres that contain the jelly can slowly give way, one by one, as exceptional loads are placed upon the system. Finally there can be insufficient fibres to withstand the pressure exerted by the central filling when it is loaded, and the disc becomes squashed. This can causes the vertebrae to come into contact enough for little side joints to be loaded. They can become inflamed with the new pressure they have to endure, and the bulging disc can irritate nerves coming from the spinal cord. In the worst case the cylinder gives way entirely, usually towards the spinal cord, as this is where its reinforcements are weakest. The central filling squeezes out like toothpaste from a tube, and presses against the spinal cord. This is the slipped disc.

It is not only the intervertebral discs that can be damaged by incautious manual handling. Muscles and ligaments can also be torn, hernial openings can be ruptured and injuries sustained from falling loads or a stumble on uneven ground. Animal connective tissue is elastic but reacts rather like plasticine or Blu-Tack® in that when cold and rested it will tear easily, but it is most pliable when warm and exercised. This is why atheletes always stretch and warm up before training and competitions. Very few emergency personnel will perform the same exercises before going on duty, but undertake more arduous exercise than they would in the gym.

SAFE HANDLING TECHNIQUE

As mentioned already, sudden unexpected movements can tear muscle, and place excessive load on the discs. The first principle of manual handling then is not to have an unexpected load. This is why the human machine's greatest strength is its brain. It can plan ahead. The long board is becoming a common feature at casualty sites. It is frequently called a spine board. The name can worry a casualty as it implies they have a spinal injury; furthermore the device is probably one of the worst things a genuine spinal injury should be strapped to for any length of time because of the high risk of pressure sores developing. It is, however, a board that can protect the spines of the rescuers. The ability to slide rather than lift a casualty has considerable advantages.

Clear the working area (including the evacuation route) of hazards in every way possible. The working platform needs to be rigid, so vehicle stabilisation needs to be reviewed. Ladders and trestles need to be secured. Check the load for anything that might prevent a secure grip. Estimate the load and decide whether to lift or slide.

The safest way to lift is the bench press. This is where the weight-lifter supports his or her spine on a bench and lifts weights above himself or herself. The shoulder girdle is therefore carrying all the load. Unfortunately this is rarely possible in the rescue scenario. The next best arrangement is to have the spine directly upright, the weight close to the spine and to lift using the powerful thigh muscles. This is the method for a carry chair lift. The feet obviously need a good solid, broad, even base. The feet should be a little more than a shoulder width apart, with one foot a little in front of the other if forward stability is required. If for any reason the footing cannot be guaranteed, or the lift throws the centre of gravity away from the spine, or it requires the spine to bend, then extra help must be considered. One of the reasons for considering a roof removal or flap on a crashed vehicle is to give the vertical height required to enable a good lifting position.

The hands should be no further apart than the width of the shoulders and the load should be spread on the whole hand rather than just the fingers. Warn the casualty that you are going to lift, as a sudden movement from the casualty can shift the centre of gravity and cause you to overbalance. The person in charge of the casualty's head and neck stabilisation is the one who calls the lift. Instructions to colleagues need to be clear, particularly when there is a group of rescuers of different disciplines. For example:

'I'm taking the head so I'm calling the shout on this lift.'

'We are going to slide the casualty up the board in several easy stages and then secure him before we lift out of the car to the rear.'

'Everybody take a secure grip. Is everybody ready?' (*Pause*)

'If we are **Ready** then – (*pause*) – **Brace** – **Slide**.'

'**Rest**. Adjust your position if necessary.'

'**Ready** – (*pause*) – **Brace** – **Slide**.'

'**Rest**,' and so on.

The use of the **Ready** – **Brace** – **Action** command is far better than **1–2–3 Lift** because helpers will never be sure whether it is 1–2– and lift on 3, or 1–2–3 and then lift, whereas the **Brace** command warns them to test the load, and the **Action** is clearly defined as **Lift** or **Slide**.

If as lifter you must bend your back from the vertical, you should try to support your upper body to replicate the four legs design. Lifting with one hand while supporting the upper body with the other will help distribute the load away from the lumbar spine. The rescue rope or fire service line can be used to help distribute the load to personnel who have secure footing and the ability to adopt an ideal posture.

The extrication of a casualty is often ill considered, all the pre-planning having been invested into the disentrapment. This is the situation where good senior officers are worth their weight. Ideally the rescue team will be casualty focused, whereas the officers will be forward planning with a team need in mind.

Figure 17.1 shows the ideal method of carrying a casualty up a steep slope. Two anchored hand lines are available to the six stretcher bearers. The downward force on the stretcher is taken by the stretcher rope. Thus the only effective moment of force operating on the stretcher is assisting the stretcher bearers to keep their footing. These lines can be laid quickly if the fire crews are requested to do so. The tendency is for this part of the rescue to be forgotten until it is about to take place. The rescuers then start up the slope with no assistance, risking injury to themselves and the casualty.

As said before, the human machine's greatest weakness is the lumbar spine, and its greatest strength is the brain. It just needs to be used.

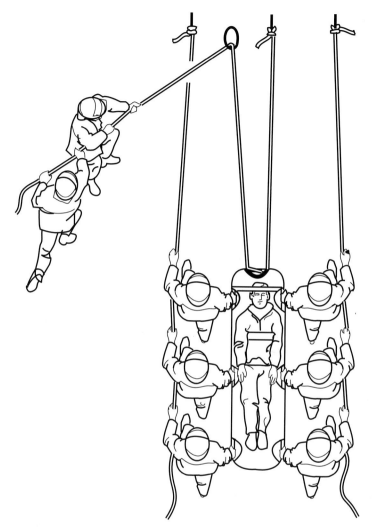

Figure 17.1   Six rescuers guide a basket stretcher up a steep embankment. They have hand lines and the stretcher is attached to its own line.

Self-test questions for Chapter 17

1. What causes muscle tears?

2. How do you avoid injury during casualty handling?

3. What is the role of the officer in charge in manual handling?

Answers on p. 215.

18

Physical fitness and safety

The emergency services have standards of fitness for their personnel and so this section has not really been written for their benefit. At the moment however there is no guidance given to immediate care doctors as to the degree of fitness expected of them if they attend an accident scene. There are many doctors who have been involved in the development of pre-hospital care in this country and are now at retirement age. There are many immediate care practitioners who have a body mass index that would class them as obese. There are immediate care doctors who suffer from illnesses that have to be notified to the Driver and Vehicle Licensing Authority.

It is very difficult to be judgemental on this issue. The doctor with 40 years of experience has a valuable resource if his or her knowledge has been kept up to date, and the doctor's driving may be superb, but is he or she fit enough to be clambering over wreckage? The police would have retired the individual, as would the fire service, and if the doctor were in the ambulance service he or she would be a senior officer on the edge of the inner cordon, or in Control. Immediate care doctors do need to get alongside the casualty, however. They cannot operate from the edge of the accident scene. They are also volunteers, and have nobody to say that they are not fit enough. Who wants to tell doctors who have been local legends for many years that they must hang up their green helmets and hand in their pagers? Once they have arrived at scene, which person will turn them away for their own safety when there is a casualty in need? The police and fire officers are in the invidious position of needing a person with medical skills at the scene, but having to allow into the environment someone whom they feel is unsafe in order to get those skills.

Good immediate care doctors are well respected, and considerable heartache is felt by people who wonder if they have to be the one to say, 'You are too overweight (too breathless, too frail, or whatever) to do the job'. As I write these words I sense that there will be people who know me, who read this book and think I mean them. I don't, but I do know that at some stage every doctor who has sacrificed his or her time and money to work alongside some of the finest of emergency crews saving lives has to make another sacrifice. The doctor has to stop – for his or her safety, the safety of the scene, and the safety of the casualty.

Self-test answers

CHAPTERS 1 & 2

1. The five stages of an accident are:
   - a failure of organisation to prevent risk factors
   - the presence of basic causes
   - an unsafe way of handling the risks
   - the incident
   - the loss to health or property caused by it.

2. Any event that has the potential for causing loss of property, loss of health, injury or death should be regarded as a 'critical incident', whether or not any such loss occurred.

3. Management can provide a safe working environment by providing **control** in the form of a safety policy that is adequately **monitored**. The possibility of a critical incident must be addressed by **emergency planning**. There must also be a protocol for **accident investigation** to enable knowledge gained from an incident to be incorporated into a reviewed safety policy.

4. Generally accidents result from one or more human failings, environmental factors or task-related problems.

5. A high-visibility jacket is essential, and an appropriate helmet with visor should be worn. A minimum of latex gloves should be worn, but hand protection may well require heavier gloves on top. Footwear should be appropriate for the terrain and spillages that may be encountered. Further protection may be obtained from a flashproof overall, and ear defenders may be necessary when cutting disc saws are used.

CHAPTERS 3, 4, 5 & 6

1. At any accident scene the principal consideration must be to the 1–2–3 rule of safety. That is, your safety is of paramount importance. Following this the scene must be made safe, and finally the casualties need to be made safe. Failing to consider risks in this order can result in further injuries occurring and possibly lives being lost unnecessarily.

2. The police will set up an outer cordon and an inner cordon at an accident scene. The outer cordon is to ensure that only those persons who have authority to approach the incident do so. This is to prevent members of the public putting themselves at risk, destroying evidence or even looting. It will also allow space for the emergency personnel to operate uncrowded. The inner cordon identifies the zone within which there is forensic evidence, casualties and risk of injury. Entry to this zone is restricted. Only personnel actually involved in the operational aspects of the rescue, and wearing appropriate PPE are permitted within the zone. They should be logged in and out of the zone. Although the police are in overall control of all incidents, the fire incident officer usually is responsible for the area within the inner cordon. He or she has the final responsibility for safety and is in command of the equipment and personnel required to effect rescue.

3. Vehicle safety is achieved by stabilisation, appropriate disconnection of the vehicle electrical system, the preparation of appropriate firefighting media for immediate use, and the institution of glass management. In the case of undeployed airbags the use of appropriate safety devices should be initiated.

4. Glass management is a concept introduced into the fire service with the intention of reducing the number of injuries caused by the material at accidents. The principle is based on the removal of glass before it breaks, or the controlled breaking of it to prevent injury from flying fragments.

5. Windscreens held in a rubber gasket can easily be removed with the aid of a stout sharp knife. A section of gasket is cut to separate the upper gasket from its lower section. The upper gasket is then pulled away all round the windscreen, which can then be removed. The procedure is described in detail on p. 28.

6. The vehicle is stabilised with step blocks and the front doors removed. Both A posts are cut parallel to and just above the sill. The front windscreen pillar part of the A posts are cut as the roof is removed. One or two power rams are the used from the bottom of the B post to the A post at dash level, or from the transmission tunnel to the dash to push the whole of the front of the car forwards. In the absence of power rams ratchet straps can be used.

7. A steering wheel relocation should never be used with an undeployed airbag.

8. Always check that the car is out of gear before the ignition is turned off in case you turn the starter motor by mistake.

9. Airbags may be identified by a small, embossed logo on the steering wheel central boss. This may say 'AIRBAG', 'SRS' or 'Supplementary Restraint Mechanism'. There may be a score line marked where the bag splits the plastic cover and there may be warning labels on the edge of the door or on the A post.

10. Casualties may be removed from being suspended by their seat belts with the long board lower. If the roof is crushed a rear oyster or side oyster may be required. Low pressure airbags can allow a lateral roof slide, and in desperation a floor pan cut may be the only option.

11. An airbag is deployed by an electrical circuit that is completed when an impact detector triggers. The detector will not trigger if the impact is more than 20° off the midline, or if the impact is less than 20 mph. If the circuit is faulty due to incorrect wiring, loose contacts, or previous damage no deployment will occur.

CHAPTER 7

1. A UKTHIS plate carries the following information:
   - Hazchem scale number
   - name of the substance and its UN code number
   - UN hazard warning label
   - specialist advice telephone number
   - symbol or housemark of the manufacturer.

2. The UKTHIS plate should be displayed to the rear and on both sides of a vehicle.

3. If there is an 'E' in the code, evacuation, or advising people to shut their doors and windows, is appropriate. Advice should be sought from the fire and police incident officers before starting this if large-scale evacuation is considered.

4. The 1–2–3 of safety is first to consider your own safety, second to consider the safety of the scene, and third to consider the safety of the casualty.

5. The fire service is responsible for the evacuation of casualties from the hot zone, and is responsible for the supervision and implementation of decontamination. The ambulance service is responsible for the care of casualties within the decontamination zone and thereafter while en route to hospital.

6. There is an International Classification System for Hazardous Materials. The classes are subdivided but the main groups are:
   - *Class 1* – explosives
   - *Class 2* – gases
   - *Class 3* – flammable liquids
   - *Class 4* – flammable solids, spontaneously combustible materials and materials that are dangerous when wet
   - *Class 5* – oxidisers or organic peroxides

- *Class 6* – poisonous or infective materials
- *Class 7* – radioactive materials
- *Class 8* – corrosive materials
- *Class 9* – miscellaneous hazardous substances.

7. The powder may give off toxic fumes that could affect the crew while within the ambulance. The latex in the gloves may react with the substance in a dangerous manner. The crew and the vehicle may become contaminated. The powder may be radioactive or a biologically hazardous substance. The casualty should therefore be held at scene until decontamination can take place there.

8. This plate is for the ADR European Transport System, which is used extensively on the European mainland. The upper number is the Kemler code and the lower number is the UN number. The Kemler code uses two or three digits to indicate the properties of the chemical. The first digit indicates the primary hazard and the next two digits any secondary hazard. An 'X' in front of the first number indicates the product does not mix with water. (Full details of the Kemler code are given in Box 7.3, p. 63.)

9. The ambulance service is responsible for the care of casualties after they have been removed from the 'hot zone' by the fire service. In the decontamination area they work in conjunction with the fire service. Once casualties have left the decontamination zone they are cared for solely by the ambulance service in conjunction with immediate care doctors.

10. Ionising radiation occurs in the form of alpha particles, beta particles, gamma rays and X-rays.

11. Radiation dose is directly dependent on the strength of the source, and the time exposed to it. It is reduced in proportion to the square of the distance from the source and to the density of the medium between the source and the individual.

12. Possible biological hazards at scene include bacteria, viruses, fungi, plants, insects, human parasites, spiders, reptiles, domestic animals, farm animals and wild animals.

13. A good first report to control would contain all the elements of an ETHANE message: exact location (E); type of incident (T); hazards involved (H); access route advised (A); number of casualties (N); and emergency services at scene and required (E).

CHAPTER 8

1. The seven rules for using a fire extinguisher are:
    1. Always summon help first.
    2. Choose an appropriate fire extinguisher.
    3. Test the extinguisher before you return to the fire.
    4. Never allow the fire between you and your exit.

5. Use the extinguisher as far from the fire as possible.
6. Never turn your back on a fire.
7. Know when to get out because the fire is winning.

2. A fire extinguisher with a black label contains carbon dioxide which is suitable for Class B fires. It will require a high concentration to put out the flames and as there is no containment this concentration will not be easy to achieve. Furthermore since the fat will be at spontaneous combustion point the flames will reappear as soon as the concentration of carbon dioxide falls below 30%. The extinguishers do not last long, the pitch of the sound of the escaping gas rising as it empties. It would be far better to exclude oxygen to fight this type of fire.

3. Since oil floats on water, the water from the extinguisher would sink to the bottom of the pan. It would then convert instantaneously to superheated steam and expand many thousand times, creating a fireball of burning oil droplets that would explode from the pan.

4. Flashover occurs when the radiated heat from a fire is sufficient to make combustible materials not directly involved in the fire burst into flame. This causes an extremely rapid extension of the fire.

5. Backdraught occurs when there is fire involving a high concentration of flammable material in a poorly ventilated and well-insulated compartment.

6. Fuel sources are classified as: Class A (carbonaceous solids); Class B (liquids and solids that melt to form liquids); Class C (gases); and Class D (metals).

7. The possibility of a backdraught should be considered if there is a lot of smoke and little flame; if the windows have oily deposits on the inside of the glass; if the door furniture is too hot to touch; if the smoke appears to suck and blow; and if the building is a modern one with double glazing or no chimneys. Whistling noises may be heard by the door.

8. BCF is an extremely potent agent that damages the ozone layer. It is also chemically altered by fire and becomes toxic to humans and animals.

9. There is the risk of backdraught, the risk of a non-respirable atmosphere, of losing your way, of being overcome, of being trapped, of being unable to extricate the casualty and becoming exhausted.

10. Foam extinguishers may use aspirated foam, aqueous film-forming foam or Alcoseal, which is resistant to methanol.

11. The dry powder extinguisher propels a blast of air in front of the powder and is characterised by an initial flare-up before the powder begins to work.

CHAPTER 9

1. Static electric sparks in an explosive atmosphere can be lethal, and receiving a hefty static shock when touching the winch line of a helicopter could cause the loss of a vital hand hold.

2. One and a half miles (approximately).

3. Lightning flowing to earth through a lightning conductor meets sufficient resistance to mean that there is ample electromotive force between the lightning conductor and any earthed object within 3 metres to create a spark between them.

4. 18 metres (20 yards).

5. 240 volts, 415 volts and 11 000 volts.

6. As an electric current flows through a circuit areas with an increased resistance will heat. If a section of the circuit is made of wire with the correct dimensions and melting point then it will allow the passage of current at the levels designed for the circuit. If the circuit is earthed, for example by someone touching part of the circuit, the current finds an easier route through the person, and the current flow is increased. This raises the fuse wire temperature above melting point and the circuit is broken.

7. The advantage of alternating current is that by passing it through a transformer the voltage and current can be changed. As the voltage increases the current decreases as the amount of energy (or number of watts) cannot be altered. A high voltage and relatively low current gives the best combination for conducting electricity over large distances.

CHAPTER 10

1. The cess.

2. You should move to the cess, face the on-coming train, and raise an arm to indicate to the driver you are aware of his approach.

3. The maximum permitted speed of trains on the line is in excess of 100 mph. Adequate clearance and refuges exist only on the opposite side of the line.

4. 9 feet (2.75 metres).

5. 25 000 volts.

6. 750 volts.

7. Even in a life-threatening emergency no part of the victim or the rescuer must be within 1 metre of the overhead line equipment.

8. Inform your control that you are going lineside. Ensure that Railtrack are aware of the situation, use signal numbers to identify precise location. If at all possible get the current switched off, or a Railtrack official to use a shorting bar. Don high-visibility clothing. Ensure one member of your party is given the task of look-out. If the current cannot be switched off use an insulated material to move the casualty clear of the line. Remove the casualty to the cess and resuscitate if appropriate. Inform control as soon as you are clear of the track environment.

9. A track circuit operating clip connects the two running rails together electrically. The automatic signalling system registers this as a train in that section and the signal to that section automatically switches to red.

10. The year of manufacture.

11. 9 inches.

12. The train's brakes are kept off by compressed air fed by a line through the length of the train. There is a valve at the front of the train with a lever that when knocked will allow the air to escape. A post beside the signal rises and lowers according to whether the signal is at stop or go. If the train passes the post when raised the lever operates and the train stops.

13. The Victoria Line.

CHAPTER 11

1. You should report to a rendezvous point (RVP). At larger airports there may be several RVPs and you should be instructed which one to proceed to. As you approach the airport there will be green signs with yellow lettering indicating the route.

2. On arrival at the main gate you should be met by an airfield air traffic controller's vehicle. You should turn off all beacons unless you have an amber airfield beacon fitted. You should follow the air traffic controller's vehicle to the incident. Do not deviate from the route taken by his vehicle. Wear appropriate high-visibility clothing; ear defenders might be necessary. When the casualty has been treated and loaded inform the airfield air traffic controller and wait to be escorted from airside.

3. Stay away from the front of an engine by a minimum of 8 metres and stay at least 45 metres away from the rear.

4. To prevent the ignition of aircraft fuel and to lay any carbon fibre fragments that could prove to be a respiratory hazard.

5. A foam blanket covers trip hazards and potholes as well as changes of level in the ground.

6. MDC is miniature detonating cord and is embedded in the perspex canopies of some fighter aircraft. It is designed to fragment the canopy moments before the ejector seat fires to permit unhindered escape. It can be detonated by a detonation cord found in an emergency access panel if firefighters need access after a crash.

7. A casualty clearing point should be at least 50 metres from the aircraft and should be in an area deemed as safe by the fire officer in command. It will usually be upwind and if possible uphill of the crash site. It should offer some degree of environmental protection. Ideally the runway and taxi routes will be used to form a one-way system for ambulances arriving and departing the loading point.

CHAPTER 12

1. The concentration of oxygen may become reduced by displacement with other gases, by fire, or by consumption in respiration. This may be countered by effective ventilation using fans or compressed air.

2. Sewer gas comprises methane, sulfur dioxide, hydrogen sulfide and trichloroethylene in variable proportion.

3. Domestic hazards are electricity, water, sewage, domestic gas, fire, chemicals, hypothermia and animals, both domestic and wild.

4. Things that might occur, indicating imminent collapse, include:
   - Sounds of creaking, cracking, crumbling or falling building materials.
   - Doors that become tight in frames while you are in the building.
   - Glass that spontaneously cracks while you are in the building.
   - Loose material that starts to fall on you.
   Other signs to note are listed on p. 140.

5. All electrical equipment must be 'intrinsically safe'.

6. Headache, nausea and confusion.

7. 'Debris crawling' is walking or crawling over the wrecked building to try to find casualties. This can cause debris to become destabilised, causing injury to both casualty and rescuer. Even if the structure does not collapse fine dust can be mobilised; this can fill voids in the wreckage that may contain live casualties.

8. Doorways, corners and edges of rooms, staircases and beside chimney breasts are all potentially survivable areas. Baths, tables and beds can also protect victims.

9. Travel tag to knots to get out.

10. STOP, breathe gently and calm down. Try to see what the problem is. If you can't, ask the person behind you to look. If there is no-one behind, tell the rest of the team ahead so they are aware of what is happening. THINK out a plan of action and then carefully try it out.

CHAPTER 13

1. No approach should be made towards a helicopter until you have been clearly signalled to do so by the pilot or other crew member. Your approach should always be via the safe route and should be while you have the attention of the pilot.

2. The no-go area of a helicopter is the entire area encompassed by the two rotors, particularly the tail rotor. The only safe approach route is directly towards the door, when the helicopter is on level ground, under direct visual contact with the pilot and at his or her command.

3. A landing area should be 15 metres in diameter with no more than a 12° slope. The approach route should be free of tall obstacles and loose debris; people and animals should be cleared over a 100 metre diameter.

4. Hundred-foot rescue ropes have tended to replace the 40-foot lashings that have been traditionally carried.

5. There are no hard and fast rules about when to rope-up. This is a decision that is influenced by a number of interrelated factors: exposure; difficulty; ability; security; the time factor; and margin of safety. (These are described in detail on p. 159.)

6. An effective roping system requires an anchor to which the belayer is secured. The belayer controls the rope to the climber.

7. The belayer needs to be able to see, or at very least clearly hear, the climber. The belayer needs to have a secure foothold. The anchor, belayer and climber need to be in one vertical line to each other, or a slip by the climber could pull the belayer off balance. The rope should not run over any sharp edges in its course.

8. Reach, Throw, Wade, Row and only then if you have to do you Swim & Tow.

9. Ropes and flotation devices can be used initially. Mudbuster boots and specialised mats can help prevent rescuers sinking. The sand lance is widely carried and is now used in conjunction with shuttering devices.

10. Strings.

11. The tide rises or falls at a given site according to the rule of twelfths (see Box 13.2, p. 163).

12. Check your knot with the diagram in the rope section. Keep practising – one day your life might just depend on your proficiency.

CHAPTER 14

1. The Course Medical Officer is responsible for the quality of the care provided at a sporting event. In the absence of a doctor being required at the event the responsibility will fall upon the most qualified paramedic or first-aider who has agreed to provide their services. As soon as someone agrees to undertake duties at a sporting event they should take steps to ensure they will be provided with the expertise, manpower and equipment that will be required. The communications with the event organisers should be documented, and if the resources are not forthcoming they should be advised in writing that you will not attend on the day of the event. The maxiumum possible notice of this should be given.

2. The Clerk of the Course is responsible for the running of a motor race circuit event.

3. As soon as any incident occurs a waved yellow flag will be displayed at the observer post before the incident. The observer post before that will

display a fixed yellow flag, and the one beyond the incident will display a green.

4. The fire marshal is indicating the need for medical assistance at the incident. It can be confused with a non-standard sign for a straight tow.

5. A marshal immediately deploys a waved chequered black and white flag before the fence. A board is placed above the fence displaying two orange circles and a chevron indicating the direction to pass the fence. Bollards will be placed across the approach to the fence.

CHAPTER 15

1. As you approach the premises try to avoid the use of blue lights and horns. Watch the windows and curtains carefully as you approach. Drive and park a little beyond the address in such a manner as to allow an easy escape. Look for signs on the door or windows that may indicate that the son has lost his temper in the past. You may wish to advise control that a police presence would be welcome even at this stage. Approach the building together, one a little behind the other. Carry a single snatch bag in your dominant hand. Knock on the door and stand to the lock side of the door. Do not enter even if the door is open but call out to introduce yourself. If the old lady calls a reply then ask where the son is before entering. If it is the son who comes to the door then assess his mood and if you feel safe ask him to lead you to the casualty. Address him as 'Sir'.

   While your partner attends to the casualty you should keep your attention on him. If further equipment is needed ask him to accompany you to the ambulance to help carry equipment. This leaves you alone with the son, but at least you are both out of the house (and have escape routes) and he is not a threat to your colleague while he is distracted by the casualty. If you suspect non-accidental injury you should not suggest that to him – indeed, all your contact with him should try to suggest that is the last thing you suspect.

   Do not refuse to let him travel with his mother, but suggest it would be easier if he came to the hospital later. If he insists on travelling ensure he is seated near the rear door, belted in position, and consider placing a large kit bag on the floor between him and you. You may use equipment from this to attend to the casualty, and it acts as a small but significant physical barrier. Inform the A&E staff of your concerns on arrival. Ensure control is aware of your concerns so they can flag the address.

2. Suspicions should be aroused if there is no reaction to your arrival or the car is parked neatly with no visible occupant. There may be unusual behaviour, for example all occupants of a car starting to approach you or the driver watching your every move in the mirror. The vehicle and occupants may appear out of place, there may be weapons visible, or the location may be a potential ambush zone. You may experience a gut feeling that all is not as it should be.

3. PPE that is in daily use at present has no protection against knife or gunshot. It is not fireproof and therefore gives no protection against petrol bombs and the majority of helmets in use have inadequate visors to cope with the hazard of thrown corrosive or ignited Class B fuels.

4. Standing disorder, running disorder and ambush.

5. Liaise with the police continually. Ambulances should be parked in secure areas behind police lines. Batteries must not be allowed to become flat. Vehicles should be parked so no single vehicle obstructs the others' ability to leave, and should always be ready for rapid retreat. Police must never be allowed to deploy using ambulances, and ambulances should travel with saloon lights on to indicate this is the case.

6. Ambulance control may be suspicious because of the nature of the call. They may however think it is a hoax call rather than a trap. The area will be usually sparsely populated but is also urban or inner city. The address itself may well be a cul-de-sac. There may be no-one to greet the vehicle or it may be a young adult keen to lead the crew to the 'emergency'. His or her body language may be inappropriate. You may notice vehicles moving to block any exit.

7. Although the appearance of letter bombs varies widely there are some characteristics that tend to show up repeatedly. Packages often have excess postage, or may have been delivered by hand and have no postage or unfranked stamps on them. They will be unexpected parcels, without a return address or a fictious address; the postmark may be different from the return address. They often have Labels such as 'Fragile – Handle with Care' or 'Rush – Urgent Package' on them. The address may be done in Letraset, or written with a distorted handwriting. There may be excessive use of Sellotape or string. Letter bombs may feel rigid, and appear uneven or lopsided in weight, while parcels may have protruding wire, aluminium foil, oil stains or even a strange odour.

CHAPTER 17

1. Muscle tears occur in muscles that have not warmed up and been carefully stretched. They occur as a result of an excessive load being applied suddenly, as occurs when either the load or the handler shifts unexpectedly.

2. If possible the casualty should be slid rather than lifted. If lifting is required the casualty should be on either a long board or a scoop stretcher. They should be secured to the stretcher prior to the lift to prevent sudden shifts of weight by their movement. The area should, if possible, be organised to allow good lifting positions to be adopted by all involved in the lift. The extrication path should be identified and cleared of hazards. The load should be assessed and adequate lifting personnel assembled. The persons lifting should operate as a team under the command of the person providing cervical spine stabilisation.

3. It is the responsibility of senior officers to ensure that the Health and Safety legislation requirements regarding manual handling are complied with in so far as is practicable considering the circumstances of the rescue. While disentrapment is progressing the senior officer should be identifying the extrication path and the evacuation route. Personnel should be deployed to clear obstacles and minimise distances. Safety ropes and other aids should be positioned. The ground should be lit if necessary. The disentrapment should be designed to permit good lifting positions to be adopted in so far as is compatible with absolute constraints. Adequate personnel need to be involved in the casualty movement. It is better that the casualty is passed along a group of personnel with good footing than a few rescuers clamber over obstacles with a casualty.

References and further reading

Department of Employment 1974 Health and Safety at Work etc. Act. HMSO, London
Department of Employment 1992 Personal Protective Equipment at Work Regulations. HMSO, London
Department of Health 1998 Guidance on chemical incidents. HMSO, London
Department of the Environment, Transport and the Regions 1999 Control of Substances Hazardous to Health Regulations. HMSO, London
Department of Transport 1989 Road Traffic Act. HMSO, London
Department of Transport 1989 Road Vehicles Lighting Regulations. HMSO, London
Department of Transport 1990 Roadcraft: the police driver's manual. HMSO, London
Health and Safety Executive 1984 Training for hazardous occupations (OP8). HMSO, London
HM Fire Inspectorate/Home Office 1983 Fire service circular 13/83. HMSO, London
HM Fire Inspectorate/Home Office 1967 – Manual of firemanship (new edn from 1999). HMSO, London
Home Office 1999 Hazchem scale card. HMSO, London
Institute of Health Service Development: Ambulance service basic training manual 1999. Institute of Health Service Development, London
Jockey Club 1999 Jockey club general instructions no. 11 (JCGI 11). Jockey Club, Newmarket
Langmuir E 1995 Mountaincraft and leadership. Scottish Sports Council, Edinburgh
London Underground Ltd: Station and track awareness for emergency services personnel, 19th edn. Railway Training Centre, White City
Rae R: A pocket guide to marshalling. Motorsport Safety Fund, West Malling

FURTHER READING

Advanced Life Support Group 1999 Major incident medical management and support. BMJ Publishing, London
Auerbach P S 1991 Medicine for the outdoors. Little, Brown & Co., Boston, MA
Burberry P 1997 Mitchell's environment and services, 8th edn. Longman Higher Education, Harlow
Eaton C J 1999 Essentials of immediate medical care. Churchill Livingstone, Edinburgh
Krebs D R 1990 When violence erupts – a survival guide for emergency responders. C V Mosby, Edinburgh
Mercedes Benz: Guidelines for rescue services 1999 Part no: 6516015802 (can be ordered from any Mercedes dealership)
Sanders M J 1994 Mosby's paramedic textbook. Mosby, Edinburgh
US Department of the Treasury website: Bomb threats and physical security http://www.atf.treas.gov/explarson/information/bombthreat/index.htm
Voluntary Aid Societies 1999 First aid manual, 7th edn. Dorling Kindersley, London
Watson L 1994 Advanced vehicle entrapment rescue. Greenwave, Halstead
Watson L 1997 How will supplementary restraint systems affect occupational safety? ResQmed, Halstead

Index